Why Not Me?

An Inspiring True Story of Survival

A tale of endurance, undying love and home made biscotti.

Why Not Me?

An Inspiring True Story of Survival

Dr. Vida Meymand

INTERNATIONAL HEALTH PUBLISHING
TAKING FORM IN A NEW WORLD

INTERNATIONAL HEALTH PUBLISHING

February 22, 2008

A Publishing Group Exposing The Truth

Cover design: Tom Meymand

Ghostwriting & Editing: Dr. Elizabeth H. Pilicy

Why Not Me? An Inspiring True Story of Survival / Dr. Vida Meymand

ISBN 978-0-9818353-0-3

Library of Congress Control Number 2008907548

SAN 856-6925

info@whynotme.tv

http://www.2GreenApples.org

Manufactured in the United States of America, and printed on the finest 100% postconsumer waste recycled paper

10 9 8 7 6 5 4 3 2 1

Dedication

I dedicate this book to my husband and my soul mate Tom. He is my backbone and the love of my life. He feeds me not only with his unconditional love and support, but also with his super delicious organic cuisine that everybody wants a bite of! He has earned the title of my "Organic Iron Chef."

Why Not Me?

An Inspiring True Story of Survival

Contents

Acknowledgments

I thank God, for loving me.
I thank my son, whom I love with a passion for continually being here for me.
I thank loved ones for supporting me.

All my appreciation and gratitude to:

Heather, for saving my life;
Our family and friends, for unlimited support;
My girlfriends, for love and time spent by my side when I needed them the most.

My special thanks to all the doctors and nurses, who helped me through my treatment as best they could.

Foreword

I am no celebrity or important somebody. I am your next-door neighbor; you may knock on my door when you are baking a cake or a pie and need to borrow a few extra eggs. I am that close to you. I am a woman just like you, and that is our bond. Let's keep our bond and beautiful network tight forever. Within these pages, my heart opens to you with my fears and sorrows, but more importantly my hope and experience of turning my nightmare into an accomplishment.

Sometimes bad things happen for good reasons. The past few years of my life initiated my personality to move through a liberating metamorphosis, like a new butterfly spreading its wings. I abolished my selfish and self-centered characteristics and dove into a deeper dimension of being I previously never knew existed. With the discovery of the depths to my own character, I now choose to live not just for myself but instead for the higher purpose of helping others.

As a woman who thought I had everything in life, I was broken to pieces by a series of events that took place one after another, all while I was waging a war with breast cancer. I reveal intimacies of how I managed to win the battle and how my eyes were opened to seeing life from a new colorful perspective.

My beloved husband Tom dedicated twenty four hours a day, seven days a week to taking care of me by cooking, washing, and pampering me. He amazed everyone with his love and devotion to his beloved wife.

In addition, I was wrapped by a delicate love and devotion from all the women I know. They never ever left me alone. I was showered by their love, spoiled by their attention. While confined to bed, I received flowers, messages, manicures, pedicures, book readings, gifts and much more. Love notes and jokes were delivered from far away, and I was supported with prayers and remarkably great energy.

No matter what happens in life, I know nothing can dissolve a bond between women because the link is bound so tightly and its network branches all over the world. I love it. Where ever we come from, whatever the color of our skin, or however old we may be – women easily connect to each other in a certain way. Women speak in a universal language to communicate with one another; women feel each other's pains and joys; women can sense if we are needed for help and rise willingly to its request. The intuitive senses exclusive to women are a foreign concept to the senses of a man.

I am an ordinary woman. I prevailed over many challenges in my life: a divorce at a young age, losing my house to a burning fire only a few years ago, no challenge so great as when I was confronted face to face by cancer. What is life without confrontation, anyway? Some people break and some people make it. Even at the lowest points in my life, I chose to make it and conquer the evils of cancer. Regardless of the nature of my challenges, I learned to build strength and carry on. Even small triumphs made me proud. By all definitions of the word, I can claim I am a survivor. But this does not make me a super-woman because the choice to survive is a choice every woman has the opportunity to apply in life. Weakness and anger have never helped anyone, so why bother?

My name is Vida – meaning "life." I decided to do just that: live and breathe life.

1

Adjusting

I was sitting in the waiting room at a county hospital full of indigent patients. The fact that I am a doctor whose practice was derailed by breast cancer made me squirm in my chair. I wore a designer jogging suit and looked as out of place as I felt. Unemployed with no insurance and a diagnosis of stage two breast cancer, I waited.

"I am a doctor, dammit. Not a patient. How did I end up here?"

Our friends and family refer to my husband and I as 'gypsies' because we have never lived in any one city for more than a few years. As a businessman, my husband loves to relocate. Our incessant moving has been the main reason preventing me from seeing my closest friends as often as I would have liked. Because of our frequent relocations, I never knew the feeling of belonging to any certain place, and never could call any of the places we lived *home*. I cannot deny there certainly *are* advantages to

1

living in various corners of the globe, such as being exposed to different cultures, seeing many new places and meeting many interesting people. However, during our continual relocations, I lost my sense of belonging; at least, this is how I felt about our endless repositioning.

Our last residence outside of the United States drastically altered my life and my attitude towards it. At a time when I needed my girlfriends the most, they were thousands of miles away across the world. I was going through menopause and the changes in my body and personality were not-at-all pleasant. If you are or have been or have known a woman in this age group, you probably know exactly what I mean. Let me tell you, I had the most severe case of menopausal syndrome any woman could have experienced. Mood swings, night sweats, and worst-of-all heart palpitations disrupted my sleep. To say it was out of control is an understatement.

The on-going insomnia cast a dark shadow over not only my physical heath, but also my personal life and business performance. Every morning I went to work exhausted before even starting my day. I mean two years of misery. Being a doctor of chiropractic, I was supposed to demonstrate top form to model for my patients and be fully capable of delivering the best care I could possibly provide. I am a strong believer in circulating karma, and wanted the best for my patients.

Despite my knowledge of what my body was going through I delayed seeing a gynecologist for advice or treatment, because I was sure the concluding verdict would be hormone replacement therapy. I was afraid of ingesting synthetic estrogen drugs into my body, and my understanding of human physiology and biochemistry fueled my fear of developing breast cancer from their use.

I've always considered myself relatively healthy: a non-smoker, a healthy diet, and an active lifestyle. I never eat fast foods or drink any soft drinks no matter how hungry or thirsty I may be. My friends often ridicule my level of extreme caution and pickiness about fat or extra carbs in my meals. My concern for my health painted an ideal picture of wellness. I assumed that having no family history of cancer, and living and eating healthy would guarantee my freedom from any disease. But life's lessons taught me no one is granted immunity from cancer.

About a year before moving back to the States, while I was still overseas I noticed a tiny dimple in my left breast at the eight o'clock position. My breast dimple did not bother me – in fact I was not surprised by it. I remembered when I was a child my mother had a dimple like this, and never had a problem whatsoever. Her breast dimple had been there as long as I could remember. Over the twelve-months after I found my own dimple, there were no changes in its size, nor any other warning signs to cause me to be alarmed.

What a fool.

Ever since my son was born, I suffered from fibrocystic breasts – a common breast condition millions of women deal with around the world. Breasts become tender and painful especially close to menstruation. With a breast sonogram, the formation of remarkable liquid-filled cysts could be visualized. The fibrotic cysts in my breasts were benign, and normally my pain and tenderness disappeared after every monthly cycle. Though less common, some women like myself have fibrocystic breasts even *after* childbearing years.

For the last year I lived overseas, I frequently suffered from pain in my left breast – mainly when I lifted heavy objects or exerted force with laboring jobs around the house. I enjoyed hobbies like home decorating and re-arranging furniture, moving things around the rooms periodically, and gardening. My friends believed I should have been an interior designer. Anyway, my breast pain increased with moderate activities, but temporarily disap-peared when I rested or took a natural painkiller.

Although I had a history of fibrocystic breasts, with breast pain and tenderness coming-and-going, the amount-ing facts that my mother had a dimple in *her* breast, there was no family history of cancer, I was a non-smoker with healthy eating habits and a relatively active daily routine, assured me I would be the last woman on the face of this earth who might be diagnosed with cancer.

"Yup. Dream on girl!"

But it was not my dimple that propelled me into action. Circumstances in my life reached a breaking point. I turned into a big monster. Did I mention I was creating a fight over any and every little thing that bothered me? I was not sure how long my husband was going to put up with my crap. The menopausal syndrome escalated to a point where it was literally ruining me. I was desperate for help and desperate to regain my life.

Well, after some time, my out-of-control hot flashes and heart palpitations finally forced me to pay a reluctant visit to my gynecologist. It took nearly six months to do so, though. Like many doctors, we don't follow the advice we give our patients.

As it turns out, when I did finally pay the dreaded visit, the gynecologist was very gentle and nice; and being a female doctor, was also very sympathetic about my personal situation.

Not having any problems her own, the gynecologist said, "I am a lucky one. Some women just do not experience any menopausal symptoms whatsoever." Before she could even consider any treatment plan for me, she asked to perform a complete check-up evaluation. She referred me for a mammogram; and being stubborn, I refused.

Yes, I am very difficult (or you may say stupid).

My defense is that mammograms have never been a sure test for either proving or ruling-out breast cancer. Being a doctor and formerly a registered nurse, I dove into any medical information I could put my hands on, and regularly researched contraindications and side effects to treatments and medications. I have read many articles detailing various cases of breast cancers that were missed even with a mammogram study. On the other hand, up to fifteen percent mammograms result in a false negative reading. Also, the procedure involves quite a bit of discomfort and subjects the breast to physical trauma each time it is performed. Because of my skepticism in the validity of mammograms, I only had a few in my entire life for baseline studies. Yes, I can see you shaking your head in disbelief. As a doctor, I felt I knew my body.

So, with my refusal of the mammogram, my doctor then ordered a breast ultrasound. The *American Journal of Radiology* reported that sonograms detect four times as many cancers as physical exams, and twice as many as mammograms. My ultrasound revealed bilateral fibrocystic breasts, with irregular borders on one of the cysts at the seven o'clock position in my left breast. The ultrasonic finding of an irregular border on a cyst was a *BIG* indication for further investigation, or in the very least a tissue biopsy. Of course, the irregularity was almost exactly where my dimple was located.

Even upon the discovery of an irregular bordered cyst, I was still not concerned about my breasts. I was in the gynecologists' office to find a way to eliminate my menopausal symptoms that drove me (and my husband) nearly insane.

If I were the gynecologist, I would not have allowed a patient to leave my office without further investigation about that breast. Because no matter who you are – a health professional or not – as a patient, you cannot think straight. Looking back, I think my desperation for fixing my menopausal syndrome distracted my doctor and discouraged her from pursuing further investigation. Otherwise, she might have insisted on searching for the cause of the problem in my left breast.

Maybe it was my destiny, though.

Whatever the reason, I have nothing against that gynecologist overseas. However, my oncologist in the U.S. did. Even my radiologist went berserk over how such an important matter was ignored without follow-up.

Truly, I think I am the one to blame, not anybody else. Because the gynecologist did indeed ask me whether I wanted to do something about the ultrasound finding of irregular tissue.

The reason she did not focus on treating the irregular bordered cyst found in the ultrasound must have been because I reacted by saying "first let's fix my menopausal syndrome."

I asked her about the possibility of breast cancer in relation to hormone therapy, and told her how I thought hormone drugs posed heath-threatening risks to hormonal balance. She agreed the chances of developing breast cancer statistically increased with the use of hormone replacement therapy (HRT). To reduce my menopausal syndrome, she prescribed Livial®, a medication with 2.5 mg per dose of the steroid Tibolone.

"This medicine is the mildest form of treatment for menopausal syndrome," she told me. "Many of my patients have seen good results by using this pill, and without any complications. The possible side effects of Livial® included a minor spotting, which should disappear in a few days," she remarked. In regards to the left breast findings on the ultrasound, though, she did not insist on any further evaluation. And since she was not firm with me, I felt off the hook!

After one week of using the pills, I began experiencing vaginal bleeding. Not just a spotting; it was a heavy bleeding. I waited for three days and the bleeding did not stop. I called her office and scheduled another appointment. Seemingly surprised by how sensitive my body reacted to this so-called "very mild treatment," she told me to immediately stop taking the pills. She also told me, I probably would have experienced even more of a harsh reaction if I *did* use the conventional HRT. Seems like my reproductive system was unpredictable; and if so, how many other millions of women are like me?

Let's assume I agreed to use conventional HRT; then what would have been the end result? I don't think it would have made me feel any better. As the gynecologist said, HRT probably would have worsened my condition.

So, here I am dealing with my hot flash and vaginal bleeding. I was back to square one, still experiencing menopausal syndrome. I asked the gynecologist what I should do? She did not have any other suggestions for me and could not help me. I was not a gynecologist to fix my own problem.

I thought to myself, "Is my only choice to deal with the misery? Hell no! I can not live my life with this." I left her office beyond upset, thinking, "There has to be something to relieve my severe symptoms."

I turned to a more natural approach, and slightly altered my diet. I decreased my consumption of coffee; and also decreased my occasional glass of wine to less than one glass per week. Those changes did not entirely resolve my problem but helped me to calm down a bit.

By then my stress levels had reached far beyond feeling helpless. Being overseas, I became increasingly homesick and blamed everything on my husband as well as the place where we were living. I started to be annoyed by everyone and everything: the climate, the lifestyle and every other little thing itched on my nerves.

While every one around me seemed to be enjoying heaven on earth, my life was becoming a living hell. I don't know whether my hormonal imbalances created the itchiness, or if it was a combination of many different issues at the time, but I wanted to return to the States.

Our family and friends envied Tom and I for living a lifestyle that appeared very desirable to them. When they realized I was thinking about moving back to the States, they thought I was crazy. Crazy to leave the luxury life we had built; crazy to close my thriving practice that was in such high demand. Because my patients raved about how well they felt after being treated, my practice was going very well. In all honesty, my patients were my only attachment. But yet again, how could I provide quality treatment when I was not feeling any good myself?

My family and friends did not know how much I was bothered by Tom's investment decisions, and the way he jeopardized his business and our bank accounts with taking risks. Tom instigated the move out of the States with his ambitious dream of earning a great deal of money overseas; however, his dream was not coming true. Despite his troubled business, he was still happy and took pleasure in seeing me at peak performance in my practice.

Worrying about Tom's business and dealing with my personal issue of menopausal syndrome made a bad combination. Truth is, I was emotionally and physically too exhausted to enjoy what other people enjoyed. All I felt was trapped in a golden cage without any fresh air to breathe. Happiness is where your heart is; and my heart was not there.

I refused to show up to public events and shied away from social exposure. What I needed was neither social stature nor flashy living. I could not find happiness there and money could not buy it for me.

Every few weeks, I reminded Tom of the reason we moved overseas to begin with – to pursue his visions of creating a unique business. He was an entrepreneur more than a businessman. At the end of the day, his interest was in creating totally new businesses that sometimes did not work out as he hoped. Our drastic departure from the U.S. was meant to be an opportunity to have an increased income from his new business venture, but ultimately only offered us a chance to work even harder. Our original plan was to spend one of our salaries while saving the second to afford us a more comfortable retirement. Nevertheless, the business calculation was not adding up.

For a stretch of time, Tom repeatedly became sick with the flu and other colds or illnesses. He stayed in bed day after day in an attempt to recover, and then was suppressed further with another episodic flu or cold. In all of our twenty years together, I had never ever seen him weak or sick. Because of his stressful worrying, his immune system was not functioning properly or adapting to the new climate.

My longing for the United States was strong, and I lobbied for us to make a move. Because we were working to only "make-a-living," our purpose of leaving the States in the first place was defeated. Our income wasn't increasing, and I simply was not happy.

I missed the little pleasures of the U.S. that filled me with inspiration: like going to local cafés with my girlfriends for lunch, or witnessing the changing of the seasons. Even my husband, who loved living overseas, admitted he missed our times spent together at *Barnes & Noble* book store café, sipping coffee and reading magazines. I took pleasure in home decorating magazines while Tom indulged in reading computer magazines.

We never managed to find a coffee shop near our house to enjoy both of our pleasures at the same time. However, there were coffee shops much fancier than in the United States, with much better tasting brews and delicious coffee bean aromas filling the air. They even served and delivered coffee to the table in real coffee mugs rather than paper cups. But no matter how good the coffee may have been, like I said, I wanted to be back home.

God answered my prayers when Tom was presented with a very attractive job offer in Connecticut. My husband was a workaholic and followed virtually every business lead. He contemplated going to Connecticut because he was beginning to realize the misfortune his investments were costing him. My husband had one month to make a decision to accept or deny the contract offer. Even though it was a short-term work offer, I still thought it was a promising financial stipend for his services. I nearly forced him to leave me to take advantage of this opportunity.

Tom was not comfortable leaving me alone to endure the misery of menopause, and not comfortable leaving me in a place I did not have family members. But I insisted, and reassured him I would be fine and would manage to wrap-up our lives overseas to move back to a place of familiarity and closer to people who cared about us.

"I can handle all the responsibility for everything here, Tom. You must go!" I insisted. This was my ticket to move back to the States. Not wanting him to have any reason to delay our move and desperate to go back home, I accepted all the duties and responsibilities and consequences. I figured by leaving everything behind we would have a fresh start. Being near my loved-ones again seemed to be the only therapy I needed to calm down and live better. The only one I would truly miss was our live-in housemaid, Padma, a beautiful soul. I relied on her one hundred percent.

Though I was aware it would not be an easy task to move our lives, I was determined and had every reason to convince Tom that moving home to the States was in both of our best interests.

With some reluctance he began his new endeavor, flying thousand of miles away, while I began shutting down our old lives to prepare for our new lives back in the U.S.

It was very difficult for me to be away from him. Especially knowing he was not within my reach. Every evening after work, I returned to the house, ate dinner in front of TV, and fell asleep. I missed Tom terribly, but was happy enough knowing I would soon be joining him in a place where I felt I belonged.

In charge of selling our house, our cars and arranging a moving company to haul our household belongings across the world, I was also handling my patients during the days and wrestling with my hot flashes and sleeplessness through the nights.

I remember Padma's sadness, crying over the thought of being left behind. We tried applying for her work visa so she could move also, unfortunately, to no avail. In my heart I knew there might be a day when she would come to the States and into our family.

Well, you can imagine the level of stress I went through to break through every impeding barrier and clear our obligations overseas in order to trail blaze our way back into the United States. Those four months were the longest months of my life.

Finally the day arrived when I was seated in the plane, Tom at my side. He came back to join me for the long flight back to the United States. Truly, I wanted to be near him more than ever. I took a long deep breath believing my obstacles were behind me, and I was on my way home.

Upon entering the United States, we spent two months in Connecticut until my husband completed his job assignment. Although within familiar territory, and beautiful as Connecticut may have been, it was just another lonely place for me and still too far away from people I knew and loved. I needed my friends close-by for comfort. I especially needed a sense of belonging.

From the moment we moved overseas until the time we returned to the States, I rode so many ups and downs, my mind and body constantly boggled by the tremendous turbulence of our circumstances and financial strife.

We talked about moving back to Dallas – where I called home. As a young adult, when I first entered the United States, Dallas was my starting point: Tom and I met in Dallas; I attended college in Dallas; I built friendships in

Dallas. So Dallas felt like my true home; and no matter how many other places I lived, deep down I always felt the need to return to the city where I had a long history. Even though Tom preferred the east coast, he graciously agreed to move to Texas to make me happy; he realized I was burnt out.

Through the sale of our house, cars and my practice overseas, we managed to generate enough money for down payments on our modest new home in Dallas and one car for us to share. The remaining funds were budgeted for our daily living expenses until we were able to earn more.

In Dallas we were like new comers because over the two years we lived overseas, society in America had changed considerably. It required time for us to re-familiarize ourselves with our surroundings and become re-established. Tom did not have anything left to invest as a business owner and job availability was slim.

The human body is design to withstand stress, but how much is too much? We could not stand for any more complexity to fall upon us. Though I didn't know it at the time, I was about to be confronted with a massive amount of stress!

2
The Eagle Has Landed

It was spring, the month of April when I boarded a plane flying east to Florida for a visit with my dearest friend Heather. She is a dentist, and is one of the nicest souls I know.

Earlier in the spring, when Heather visited Dallas to spend time with her parents, I received a call from a mutual friend informing me Heather was in town. Tom and I had only been in Dallas two weeks. Exhilarated to learn she was in town, I wanted to have the chance to catch a visit with her. Heather's mother and I also have a very special relationship; she always treats me as if I am her own daughter. Between the three of us we share a very close connection that exceeds an average friendship. Even throughout the years when I lived abroad, the distance did not loosen the strength of our ties. Many years had passed since we last saw one another.

Let me rewind to even earlier in the spring, about two weeks before Heather's visit to Dallas when my husband and I were out of town for business purposes. He completed his work assignment a few days earlier than originally planned, so we returned to Dallas a few days sooner than scheduled. This change of plan provided the opportunity for me to see my dear friend Heather, whom I had not seen for many years. This is a long story, and I will reveal just how coincidence was capable of changing or perhaps even saving my life.

As soon as I gained knowledge of Heather being in town, I called her right away. Hearing each other's voices through the phone, we both became emotional and sentimental.

"My flight back to Florida is in a few hours." She said, unaware I had returned from my trip.

"I'm in Dallas,!" I informed her. Changing her flight schedule to stay any longer was not possible because her dental clinic opened early and she needed to leave in time to be there the next morning for her patients.

I offered her a ride to the airport so we could have some time to spend together. I hung up the phone, quickly rushed from the garden where I was watering the flowers back inside the house, grabbed my keys, jumped in my car and drove to pick-up Heather.

I cannot describe the excitement of seeing each other after so many years. We held each other, hugging, crying joyfully. There were only a few hours to be with her before her flight departed, and with so much to catch up on and talk about.

At that time I had a nagging chipped tooth. As we drove to the airport, I told her about the chipped tooth and asked her what to do.

"Take an x-ray and have it sent to me," she recommended. I am a chicken when it comes to dental offices. I am sure I am not the only one scared of the sounds of drilling.

About a week after Heather departed, my local dentist took an x-ray and said my tooth was broken; and since there was an adjacent crown, the chipped tooth could not be saved. It needed to be extracted. The only option left for me was an implant. I was not pleased with this news; the last thing I wanted to do was to have a tooth implant. I just did not like the concept.

I asked the dentist to e-mail the x-ray to Heather in Florida. Heather had been my main dentist as long as I can remember. I flew from where ever I lived in the country to see her for my dental work. Maybe because she has a tender loving touch the extra travel was never a bother.

Besides, not only was she one of the best dentists I could ask for, she was one of my closest friend.

When Heather reviewed my dental x-ray, she called me.

"I can save your tooth. Come to Florida. You can stay with me, like old times." When Heather invited me to spend time with her, I seized her offer.

"Ahh Florida." I relaxed into my seat on the airplane. I thought, "Soon I will land to have fun with my girlfriend and fix my broken tooth, all on the same convenient trip." I was excited to be going to Florida.

As I was flying, I thought back to the year 1992, when Tom and I were still living in Florida. Heather and I were inseparable; going out for lunch was our special get-together event. We ate lunches at different places each time, but our ultimate favorite spots were South Beach and the eloquent Bal Harbour near Miami. Sometimes she drove up to the beautiful small town of Boca Raton where I used to live. The sidewalks outlined by restaurants, elegant boutiques and delightful coffee shops – all for the two of us to enjoy. The light breeze off the ocean's shore cooled us while sipping at our coffee, chit chatting. I still remember as if it were yesterday.

Heather and I spent hours deep in conversation about the latest best selling books. We took pleasure in discussing non-fiction literature, the plots and character developments in the books; we loved reading about people. The two of us maintained a multi-dimensional relationship spanning from being foxy gals on the hunt of fashion, to spiritual enthusiasts. We both highly value being in touch with our beliefs and our communities. Heather's spiritual side devotes much time and energy to helping others in every way she can, including financially.

I adjusted my posture in my seat to look out the window of the airplane. Leaning forward, I gazed at the sky's horizon. I remembered the weekends when Heather and I collaborated with the rest of our families and she played her guitar while I sang along. Heather's great sense of humor and silly little jokes make people laugh out loud. We both love shopping and occasionally we "shopped 'til we dropped."

A most memorable day was when I told her about my plan of moving to Texas for enrolling in school again. We were eating lunch at one of our favorite spots, when I told her I planned to study to become a doctor of chiropractic. Heather did not like the idea of me leaving Florida. I totally understood; the idea of moving away from each other was as difficult for me.

"Here's a plan: I will offer you total financial support for one year if you stay and open a design center in Florida." Her light-hearted idea sprang from her lips. She always admired my interior decorating style. Still, I always aspired to become a doctor and was destined to make it a reality. As a deeply close friend, she was entirely supportive of my pursuits and said she was certain I would become successful.

Ever since I was a little girl, I was interested in being a doctor, and played around the house with my siblings pretending to treat their scrapes and bruises. My mother was a pharmacist and extremely reliant on the miracle of what medicine could perform! As a child, my dislike of taking pills that sometimes was mandatory from my mother gave me a taste that still is to my dislike.

How could I become a doctor without caring for medicine?

I became a registered nurse and worked for a few years as a scrub nurse and planned to go to medical school when an event sent me in a life changing direction. A car accident in 1991 caused two disc bulges at the lower level of my cervical spine. Pain was unbearable and I was crying when Tom drove me to the hospital. I experienced numbness and tingling in my fingers and lost about thirty percent of my strength in my left arm. That experience taught me compassion for patients who lived in pain. The neurologist in the hospital suggested surgery for the condition of my neck.

From my background as a nurse, I was fully aware of the possible side effects and risks involved with surgery. I decided to seek a second opinion. In my search for another doctor, I visit a chiropractor that was recommended to me by a friend. Feeling as though I had nothing to lose, my expectations of the chiropractor were nothing more than conducting an investigation to his opinion.

I started a course of treatment. One week of chiropractic treatment and my pain level decreased tremendously. After two months of treatment, my strength in my arm fully returned. In addition, I could sleep, I could move more freely and my pain was diminished in most parts. My interest in chiropractic was sparked, and the option of becoming a doctor without having to rely on prescription medication matched my personal beliefs about healing. As a Chiropractor, I have been working with reputable orthopedic surgeons and neurologists. We refer patients to each other when it is necessary.

As the morning sun shinned on me through the small oval window next to my seat in the airplane, I remembered how difficult it was to say good-bye to Florida when I started chiropractic school. In order for me to pursue my dream of becoming a chiropractor, Tom and I had to leave our very pleasant and comfortable Florida lifestyle, and Tom had to liquidate his successful business. Other than when Tom and I moved from overseas back to the States, as I mentioned, moving out of Florida was the only other time in our marriage I initiated a transfer. Any and all of the other zillions of times we moved from one state to another, or one country to another were Tom's business moves. Supportive of my decision to become a doctor, he believed in me and still does to this day.

I was deep into my own thoughts when the flight attendant announced our landing into Miami. The entire flight seemed to me like a New York second! My girlfriend Heather picked me up during her lunch break and we drove straight back to her dental clinic to start my dental work. Knowing I had a deadline to return to Dallas in order to continue on flying overseas for business, there was no time to waste and Heather wanted to make sure all of my dental work could be taken care of prior to my departure.

After much drilling, Heather and I went to lunch and wanted to graze over years of talk in the first day of my arrival. It was so amazing to realize true friendships never fade, even with being apart for numerous years. It seemed like only yesterday – going out to lunch as we used to, and we could not feel even a slight gap of time or space between us. We had a wonderful time together, we always did. I felt my emotions stirring when I saw her young children grown up and gorgeous. Heather's husband, Sam has always been like a brother to me. I really felt so very happy to be visiting with their family again.

The second day of my visit with Heather, we had the chance to go out to the shopping boutiques. We spent quality time talking, naturally.

That evening, Heather came to the guest room where I was about to tuck in for bedtime and knocked on the door to say good night. Again, we started talking, this time about fashion, new trends in style and cosmetics – as most girlfriends carry on. As she was sitting on my bedside, I realized there was a little scar on her skin at her waistline.

"What happened there?" I asked her about her little scar.

"Minor surgery," she said.

I lifted my shirt showing her my little dimple on my left breast.

"This is my natural scar, but I'm not worried about it because my mom has one, too!" I said.

She thought I was insane and shocked me as she began yelling and shouting.

"You are telling me that you have not checked that out? And you call yourself a doctor? Don't you realize that could be an indication of breast cancer?" She then started questioning me, "How long have you had this dimple on your breast?" Her concern was if it was cancer causing the dimple, perhaps it might have spread to various other parts of my body. Then she accused me of being too spiritual and looking forward to dying and going to heaven to join God.

"Well…" Taken-back by her reaction, I did not really know what to say to calm her down. I tried to assure her. "As soon as I return to Dallas I will have it checked out."

She said she did not trust me. "If you care about this dimple, you would take it more seriously." Heather started to interrogate me again about when it started and what happened. "When was the last time you had a breast evaluation?"

"Well…" I began telling her everything from 'A' to Zimbabwee: the mood swings, the heated flashes of sweat dripping in the night, the pain – on, off, and on again. I told her of the complacent doctors overseas, the cysts, the pills, the bleeding, and how my exhaustion and menopausal syndrome were major influences on my decision to move back to the States. By the time this conversation came to a close, it was well after two in the morning.

"Goodnight Heather." I was mentally exhausted.

"Goodnight." The tone in her voice told me she was more than upset.

Heather awoke the next morning on a mission to have my breast checked. She made several brief telephone calls to arrange an emergency appointment for me with two different clinicians. From her abrupt actions, I started to worry and wonder if there was really something wrong with me.

After one day in Florida, I had a mammogram of both of my breasts, followed by a breast ultrasound. We were literally rushing from one clinic to another. Heather was so nervous and worried that she was unable to hide her sincere concern. The next few days we sat idle waiting to receive the results.

What was the verdict?

If I told you I was still not concerned after talking with Heather, I would be lying. For the first time, I *was* truly worried. No matter how hard we both tried to stay calm and conceal the overflowing thoughts as we gauged the odds, we could read the troubled looks on each other's faces. Even then, she was still more apprehensive than I. Too optimistic, I simply did not want to accept the probability or likelihood of anything severely wrong with my breast and it's dimple.

It was a Saturday afternoon, two days after all the rushing from clinic to clinic. Heather and I were shopping in a home accessory store when Heather's cell phone rang out from her designer purse. I didn't take much notice because first of all, it was *her* purse ringing, not mine. And second, who would call on a weekend about a diagnostic test result, any way?

As you might have guessed, the doctor in charge of my case was calling to notify her of the results of my mammogram and ultrasound, as Heather had requested a prompt response. I was wrong about the weekend. As a friend, the doctor did a favor and placed his follow-up call on a Saturday: a phone call that changed the course of my life.

I was still looking for decorative items for Heather's house when I saw her talking into the phone and then she turned her face toward me. I saw angst in her demeanor and crinkling in her otherwise beautiful face. She could not mask anything from her dearest friend. We made eye contact, her look conveying what was said in the telephone conversation. I was motionless and unable to move, inoperative. She ran towards me with uncontrollable tears streaming down her cheeks and embraced my fear with her arms around me. We held each other tightly.

There is not a word, a phrase or even a book that could elucidate that most painful moment of doom. I tried very hard to refute my feelings of horrified emotion. I tried even harder to pacify the situation by staying composed. God only knew what was going on inside me. No words in any language explained the storm raging through my mind, my heart, and my soul.

"Oh my Lord, is this a bad dream? It cannot be happening to me! What am I going to do?" I thought, "How am I going to tell Tom? What about my son?" Shawn was coming to see me at Heather's for two days before my return home. "What about my parents?" Neither was in good health. "How can they handle this devastating news? What about the rest of my family and friends?" I was flooded by a down pour of worry.

I felt like a criminal who did something terribly wrong, like breaching everyone's faith in me. I felt like a victim, robbed of my vitality. Why was Heather the one to go through all of this grief with me? Our pain was all because of me. A doctor, and I failed to identify the most threatening disease of my entire life. I began riding the proverbial emotional rollercoaster and without any control, it took me to the crest of its scary heights and dropped me all the way down to the very bottom. I was numb.

As the last few days of my stay in Florida elapsed, I felt as if I existed in a foggy space, everything around me cloaked in a clouded and delusional film disabling me form seeing or feeling reality. With all I was going through, I tried to stay tough and provided emotional support to Heather. She constantly scrolled through websites on the Internet, collecting as much information as she could possibly gather to help me. I rested and slept while she searched endlessly for answers. I wanted to shut down my entire system to escape fear and confusion.

Under the covers of exhaustion, I fell asleep soon after I lay down each night. A stranger to relaxation, I woke up in the darkness unable to fall back to sleep. Unsure of what was going to happen to me, I wondered if cancer had crept throughout my body. My thoughts were dull and my mind went blank. As strong as I thought I was, I could not think clearly and could not make any deductions of my predicament.

"This was supposed to be my 'little vacation.' I was planning to have fun with my girlfriend." I sank deeper into disappointment.

"What is going on?" I thought more, with no answers. Nothing was predictable at all.

While we waited for my son to arrive, Heather's husband Sam took us out in his fishing boat for a day on the Gulf cruising. Every effort was made to keep me busied, and they entertained me every which way imaginable to distract the reality of what I was facing. I decided it was best to have a good time with them while I was there, not letting the time be wasted by worry. Like the saying goes, "Why mourn for a death that has not happened?"

"Let's enjoy life!" I said to myself. "For at least today."

We all enjoyed the ocean and our surroundings.

That evening my son Shawn finally arrived. I had no idea how I would tell him; but since he did not yet know anything, we all put my diagnosis in a box that would stay unopened for the night. By boat, we went to dinner at a Cuban water front restaurant and I made the best of every minute with Shawn and my loving friends. Spending an evening with everyone by the beautiful coastline truly helped me to block out my emotions. At the restaurant, the waiter helped Sam tie up the boat, grabbing the ropes as we scooted in towards the dock. We sat by the patio facing the ocean. I took-in the misty air as needed breathes of life, facilitating the amazing ability to lead and coach my mind from sadness to happiness.

We retired back to Heather and Sam's late in the evening. I decided to wait until morning to disclose my devastating news to Shawn.

After breakfast, Shawn and I went for a walk in the garden, strolling arm-in-arm through the flowery bushes and plants. We then sat on the pool deck, talking about his life. I scavenged the back of my mind for a way to bring my shocking news into the conversation. Until then, I had not truly recognized the dexterity required to unveil distasteful news to a loved one. I did not know where to begin. I kept asking him questions and buying time in anticipation of being ready to talk about myself.

"I have something very serious to tell you, Shawn." I finally found the courage to tell him about my diagnosis and tamed my emotional side.

He held me next to his chest and said, "I will stand by your side, Mom." With his embrace enveloping my dread, I could no longer suppress my dismay and began crying uncontrollably. I did not know where all my tears were coming from.

"I'm very scared," I told him. "I'm so disappointed and angry with all of this. I am so angry!" I muttered between my streaming tears. I could not believe how supportive he was for me. He made me feel so loved and at ease with his calming warm hugs and gentle kisses to my forehead. A relief to have Shawn by my side, I was thinking of the other man I loved so much, Tom, and how far away I felt from him.

The next day I actually felt much better and I promised Shawn, "I will never disappoint you; and I will fight the cancer with all of my might and all of my mind power."

The last day of my stay in Florida, we made a video of Heather playing the guitar while I sang along – just like the good old days when we lived a few miles away from one another. We sang a concert of prayers for a successful recovery for me, and celebrated our loving memories. Basically, we did whatever we could think of to stay upbeat and cast negativity far out to bay.

As Shawn was leaving for Daytona Beach where he lives, we said good-bye to one another.

"I love you, Shawn."

"I love you too, Mom. I will come to Dallas to support you. Let me know when you will be having your surgery. I want to be there for you." He waved good-bye as I watched him until he was no longer in my view.

3

The Universe's Healing Energy

To prevent even one hour from going to waste, Heather changed my airline ticket for an earlier flight back to Dallas to speed up the necessary arrangements for my treatment back home. I was not sure how my husband would handle the news about me. How could he possibly accept his strong and healthy wife was returning home diagnosed with breast cancer? I did not know what to do.

My husband and I are soul mates. All our family and friends admire our endearing love for one another. Despite so many ups and downs – probably equal to the turmoil every relationship experiences – we managed to survive and keep our love intact and growing. My friends have often asked me how I uphold a loving relationship with Tom, and if we ever have any sour moments in our marriage life. One day when I have free time, I shall write a book about 'how to handle a husband,' or in other words, 'how to keep love alive.'

Tom and I first met in a club in Dallas, when I was just recovering from my divorce. Interestingly enough, he was also recovering from his recent divorce. The last thing on my mind was commitment. However, I started dating him occasionally, just wanting to have fun, nothing serious. Then we began realizing our relationship had developed into something much stronger than a desire for dating. We fell in love, and after two years sealed our love in marriage.

Over twenty years ago when we married, we promised we would be together "for better and for worse, 'til our death do us apart." We actually practice our oath. We never attempt to change each other because the reason we fell in love from the start was the admiration we had for one another as we were. Sticking together and accepting one another have been the touchstones for our successful marriage.

The day after I was diagnosed, I asked Heather to call Tom over the telephone to allow time for him to absorb the news while I was still away. She told him all about what he did not want to hear. I cannot imagine how tough it was for her to tell him the bad news. After Heather brought him up to speed, Tom and I talked over the phone briefly, but he shied away from talking about my breast cancer; he sounded strong. He told me how much he missed me and wanted to have me home next to him. We did not have any discussion about my diagnosis. Since he did not have the heart to bring up the subject of cancer, I decided to wait until I was back home.

After Tom found out, he went to Heather's mom's house in Dallas and shared the painful news with her, crying like a baby on her shoulder. Like me, Tom is very close to Heather's mom. She is a timeless soul, one of many good friends we are blessed to have in our lives.

Flying back home, I was not looking forward to my arrival and did not want to face anything or anyone, especially my husband. I wished I could walk home instead of flying so I would not arrive so soon. Realizing I had to go to the hospital and deal with reality, I was not ready for anything at all.

My husband picked me up at the airport; it seemed like years we had been away from each other. He met me at the end of the terminal, and we walked to the car with hands held so tightly nothing could tear us apart. On our way home, I showed off my brand new tooth and how great it looked. I told him about everybody in Florida: Sam's fishing boat, our son's visit, and the celebration with the guitar and singing concert-movie, and much more. We talked about everything except cancer. We didn't want to ruin our precious moments together by discussing sad news.

Like everything else, there was an end to the show and reality had to be faced no matter how difficult it might be. After only one day with Tom, I began to observe how sensitive he was to discovering his wife's diagnosis of a terminal illness. I needed to have an important conversation with him. I knew how much he loved me and how emotionally dependent he was on me.

"Tom, the only way I can go on to fight cancer is with you staying strong and positive for me." He listened closely and had a compassionate look in his eyes. I told him the same thing I said to Shawn. "I promise I will not disappoint you." His eyes lit up with hope as I said, "I will live by your side for a very long time! There are people out there who die of heart attacks or sudden accidents or other unexpected events; but I'm alive! So let's celebrate life; that is why we have been born."

Over the course of the first week of my diagnosis of breast cancer, as hard as the news was continually hitting me, I never asked God, "Why me?"

I thought to myself, "If not me, then who? Do I know any body else I'd want to suffer in my place?" I truly couldn't think of anyone, so "why me?" wasn't even a valid question.

I continued my rationalizing thoughts, "why *not* me? Is my blood any thicker than any other women out there?"

Like I said, I am an ordinary woman; I *know* that. In the recognition of being just like other women, I came to peace within myself.

With a little time, Tom was also feeling much better. He saw in me a sense of control over the situation, and a sense of straightforwardness, as if I could persevere. My willpower and inner peace helped not only my husband, but also the rest of our family and friends to relax and avoid becoming overwhelmed by my disease.

Having said there was peacefulness about us, every now and again I fell into candid 'Kodak' moments where repressed emotions clutched at the better part of me. However, with great effort I cut the crying rampages short and clutched back at getting a grip. Refusing to let worries and bad images take over my mind, I cleared my thoughts of any of the so-called normal terrors that come with an unexpected diagnosis of disease.

My silly little secret I share with you: during the sad moments, I sat in front of my vanity mirror and talked to myself out loud.

"Are you done crying? Look at yourself! What happened to Miss Positive? Didn't you say you would be strong?"

Then I repeated over and over, "I am healthy. I am healthy. All the healing energy in the universe is coming towards me to help me heal. Accept this energy."

Since crying brings negative energy, it conflicted with universal healing powers that echo vibrant positive energy. So in order for me to receive the universe's healing energy, I had to stop crying. I even made silly faces in front of the mirror to make myself laugh really hard. Pretty much, I became my own clown and emotional therapist. It was working, though. Soon after this practice, I reached the point where I barely cried over anything, even things that had previously paralyzed me with tears.

I cannot emphasize the power of the mind. Hearing ones own voice speak positive phrases is auto-suggestive encouragement and resonates in our beings. Controlling the mind requires a focused direction of thought and convicted belief; it truly works at creating an optimistic outlook. I understood the tension of being wound up; but I learned how to deal with all of my tension and pain by talking myself through the mud.

Back in Florida, the doctor recommended a biopsy, which is a further diagnostic procedure after a mammogram and ultrasound to help the Oncologist find out more about the type of the tumor. I waited until I returned to Dallas to follow through with the biopsy so Tom would be with me. I needed his loving tender touch more than ever.

All of the procedures I needed were going to be extremely expensive, and I thought about the ways I planned to afford to be treated. I have never had health insurance in my life. I was always healthy and assumed I would remain healthy.

"Why should I waste my money on paying insurance bills? For a woman like me, a self-employed doctor, it does not make sense to throw away my money by paying for high priced insurance every month." Insurance was not a priority.

Other than the prescribed Tibolone steroid for my menopausal syndrome that left me with severe vaginal bleeding and reinforced my belief that I was better off without medication, I did not use prescription medications. Instead, I subscribed to and endorsed holistic healing. The only pills I ingest are vitamin and mineral supplements. Subscribers to health insurance policies are not reimbursed even a single penny for buying nutritional supplements. The only wellness compensation I can think of is the willingness of some insurance companies to co-pay for health exams or a reimbursement for an activity center membership fee, and that is if the health plan is with a quality provider. Knowing what I know today and considering all pros and cons, would I invest in health insurance?

I probably would. If one can afford insurance, having its benefits is an enormous security for desperate situations, like mine. Because insurance companies will not provide coverage for patients with disease and they reject applicants with pre-existing medical conditions, the likelihood of being insured after being diagnosed is very slim.

I had no insurance, I was unemployed and my condition left me three choices: do nothing, pay out of my pocket, or turn to the county hospital. I wanted to live and I could not afford the massive expenses of breast cancer treatment. My time was running out; the only realistic choice I had was to go to the county hospital.

With research, I discovered the local county hospital had an association with the local medical university. Well known and well respected, the hospital utilized state of the art diagnostic and medical equipment and offered many great programs to under-financed patients.

After my admission to the county hospital, the receptionist sent me to the oncology department. To keep calm and center myself, I meditated the night before and just prior to going to the hospital. Tom and I walked hand-in-hand along the lengthy hallways of the crowded hospital following arrows and signs on the walls to find our way.

I thought, "Is this me going for oncology?" It was very hard for me to accept the fact that I was seriously ill. I entered to the reception area and saw bald and very pale women sitting and waiting.

"My God, why am I here? Am I really sick or is this a very bad dream?" I was not used to sitting in a waiting room to be treated.

"My job is to *see* patients, not to *be* a patient," I thought. Yet my days as a doctor adjusting patients seemed as far in the past as the clinic I left behind me.

They asked me to change into a hospital gown and wait. With his arm around my shoulders, Tom comforted me with the promise of stirring up his delicious lentil soup as soon as we returned home. He always filled the emptiness of the waiting period with conversation and support; there was love in the air when ever he was with me.

After about forty minutes, a group of doctors called me in for a detailed physical exam and case history, then more waiting with Tom.

The group of doctors walked over to us where we were seated and called us back into a room to report a confirmation that the tumor in my breast was malignant. I remained unusually calm and asked questions about my case.

"What do I do from here on?" Our meeting was a general observation of my case, and we set a plan for the pre-operation procedures. The hospital discarded the mammogram and ultrasound performed in Florida and scheduled me for both tests again.

"We do not want to be responsible for any misdiagnosis of any kind, so we will be taking some more images." The medical doctor explained.

After the bilateral breast ultrasound, they scheduled me for a core needle biopsy.

At eleven o'clock in the morning, I arrived to the radiology department with my husband. Three other women sat staring at the walls in the waiting room. A woman deep in thought caught my attention. She was in her thirties or so, and waited quietly by herself. Nobody else was talking, so I decided to split the stale air by starting a conversation with her.

"I have breast cancer, how about you?" I asked.

"I was misdiagnosed by my gynecologist," she said. "They don't even know how far the cancer has gone. I'm late for work; I just want to leave now." I heard a nervous tone in her voice.

I told her not to worry, and reminded her about all the new medicines and advancements in technologies.

"Don't worry too much." I said offering hope to her, but also, perhaps I was reassuring myself at the same time.

The attendant that called out my name showed me to a room where I could replace my clothes with a hospital gown. Then, I was led to the biopsy room. A radiologist walked in and explained the procedure. I did not mention anything about my occupation as a doctor.

"When you are the patient, act like one." I said to myself.

Thanks to the newest technology, the performing doctor found the exact location of the lesion and marked it before any needle entered my body with no guesswork involved. I could see the route of the needle across the computer screen.

The doctor's assistant was in such a bad mood I could feel a negative vibration bouncing all around the room. She continually complained about being tired.

"They asked me to stay over-time again, and I don't want to today...I can't do it." She announced to everyone.

To say the least, the room's atmosphere was thick with intensity. Lying on the biopsy table, I watched the assistant in front of the computer at my right side control the mouse on the screen to aid the doctor during the procedure. Then, I looked back to the doctor working on my left breast, and back to the computer screen where he looked while inserting and guiding the biopsy needle through my skin into my breast towards the lesion. The core biopsy needle, large enough to hold a tiny cutter at its tip, reached the tumor and the doctor instructed the assistant to push the start button. The device connected to the biopsy needle was enabled and the doctor removed a sample of tissue from my breast. The local anesthesia numbed me from feeling any pain during the biopsy.

I smiled at the assistant, but it did not transform her disposition in any way; she was extremely upset about working overtime. It seemed like my bad day should have trumped hers.

My frustration with her made me want to post a complaint with the head doctor about her unprofessional behavior. But something inside me prevented my anger from escalating. Focusing inwardly, I convinced myself that whatever was happening in the room on that particular day, must have held a lesson for me to learn.

So instead of protesting against her attitude, I asked, "Are you alright?"

"No I am not alright," she replied. "I am tired!" It seemed as if the doctor in charge was afraid of her; perhaps she had been working there for a good long time.

"You must be having a really bad day," I assumed. "Just take a few deep breaths and before you know it, you will be going home."

She kept her silence for a moment before spilling her built up tension.

"I have a plateful. My father is sick and we have a strong bond and His illness is killing me. My only son is a Marine, fighting in Iraq and I'm not even sure I will ever see him again. Now here I am: hungry, tired, and forced to stay at work because the supervisor told me to."

"We all have bad days, but soon everything will be okay," I replied. To my surprise she started smiling back at me and came to my side to start working without any more anger. She even held my hands to comfort me during the remainder of the biopsy procedure. Even though I thought I was mentally prepared by my meditations, the biopsy procedure was extremely stressful for me. I was quite familiar with the procedure from my days as a nurse, but this time I was the patient and pretty much rendered helpless.

"Sweetheart, it will not take too long and you will be free to go!" She told me. I was amazed by how my little anecdote of sweetness changed her attitude from being angry at the entire world to being a sincerely caring person.

After my biopsy was completed, with gentle approach she said, "Let me give you a hug." As her arms reached around me, she said, "Thank you for not judging me. I am not always this nasty."

The idea of handling the intense situation in the biopsy room with tenderness was the kind of way I began helping myself forget about my own pain and fear. Perhaps that lesson was one I was meant to learn through the process. I felt so good about how I handled the awkwardness. It was a breakthrough moment. For the first time in my life, I was not self-centered and demanding. As a patient, I had every right to complain about the assistant nurse and her demon-strative reaction in front of me. As vulnerable as a cancer patient could be, the biopsy room was not an appropriate place for a nurse to be complaining.

Then I started questioning, "Is this how cancer changes someone? The way I feel myself changing?" If so, I was actually looking forward to seeing even more productive changes in myself along the road. The day of my biopsy was when I realized everyone has the potential to make a difference in people's lives.

4
Apple Green Pajamas & A Candle of Hope

One week after my biopsy, I received a call from the hospital. Although I already knew the diagnosis from the doctors back in Florida, I was still hoping for the slight possibility there had been a mistake. Hope is such a powerful tool. However, the result of my ultrasound and biopsy was the confirmation of a malignant tumor in my left breast, just as the ultrasound taken in Florida revealed and just as the doctors told me after my physical exam. The week preparing for surgery was the longest week of my life.

Immediately upon being notified of the confirming diagnosis, I was scheduled to see a surgical oncologist: a breast cancer specialist. When I went for my appointment, I filled out the paperwork at the front desk. Then, I waited for quite a long time before they sent me into an exam room.

I saw a young mother holding her infant slouched in a wheelchair being pushed by a nurse. Her skin was pale and somehow dehydrated. They were rolling towards the chemotherapy room. My heart ached at the sight.

I thought, "God, am I sick and in this hospital for a certain reason? What is the purpose for me to have to go through this physical and emotional trauma?" I wished I had a truck-load of money to take care of all those cancer patients.

"I am poor myself, otherwise I would not be here." I realized. "I know our poor financial situation is not going to stay like this. Sooner or later we will stand tall again. My mission is to rise to these challenges. Then I have a mission and that is why I have cancer and that is why I am in this county hospital." I set my attitude for the day, and continued, "I have to do something to make a difference. God please help me. Let me leave a good footprint before my time is over." I felt entirely responsible for the people I saw in that hospital, as if I had a bountiful bank account or something else to offer to them. "How can I help them?" I kept asking myself.

Once I was in the exam room, I waited again for the surgeon. My husband was with me the whole time and never left my side. The nurse checked my weight, my vital signs – heart rate, blood pressure, and pulse all over again. My anxiety was building and was not helped by the discomfort of being in a freezing cold exam room.

As an aside, I suggest bringing along a sweater or something to keep warm while waiting in a hospital. Even for testing or screening procedures, an extra warm sweater comes in handy. If you have never been to a hospital and go for the first time, everything may look completely foreign. It's a cold and sterile environment. It is best to arrive a little earlier and plan time for navigating through the hallways to find the department of destination. Every little hint I offer here may be helpful for feeling in control and eliminating unnecessary anxiety. As a doctor, I was no stranger to hospital corridors and exam rooms; however, as the patient the setting felt unfamiliar and somehow strange.

Finally, my assigned surgeon walked in with a nurse practitioner that I had met previously. A second nurse unknown to me followed in behind them. Come to find out, this nurse was a living angel and did everything in her power to help me; truly she made a difference and I will always remember her kindness and helpfulness towards every one around her. The nurse practitioner, the one I knew previously, was very knowledgeable and well experienced in his field. He also was wonderful and helped me to the best of his ability.

Surprisingly, a young attractive female doctor also came into the exam room. Shortly after she arrived and cordially greeted me, our personalities clicked. My anxiety level dropped next to nothing. I could not have asked for a better team of medical personnel; they gave me a comfortable feeling of relief.

The doctor examined my breasts, feeling the tissue with her fingertips. Because I had undergone so many different tests and diagnostic procedures, not to mention observations and palpation examinations, my breast was fairly sore. I never imagined the day when mine would be more scrutinized than Dolly Parton's boobs.

My surgeon gave me two options for my breast surgery. The first option was a radical and total mastectomy of the affected breast, which would exempt me from radiation therapy. The second option was a lumpectomy, meaning they would remove the lump and some of the surrounding tissue, but leave my breast intact. The second option would be treated with radiation therapy; we had not yet determined if chemo was needed or not. Prior to the surgery, there was no way of knowing the exact size of the tumor or if my lymph nodes were involved. My entire treatment plan would be determined after the consideration of the results from the surgery and pathology findings. I decided to have the lumpectomy, even though I would have to undergo radiation therapy. I did not mind going for radiation therapy every day if it could save my breast.

My surgeon said, "We can only determine what your needs are when we dissect the breast. There are a few more tests required before your surgery." The surgeon ordered a bone scan, a complete body scan, a blood panel, and a heart scan.

"A few?" I thought.

"You should avoid eating soy products just in case the tumor is estrogen sensitive," the nurse practitioner suggested. For years I drank soymilk and other soy products on a regular basis, mostly because soy was said to be a source of carcinogenic fighting agents.

We live, we learn.

With a disease like cancer – feared by all – it is so easy to panic and become lost. The best approach for a patient is to conduct research and collect as much data and information as possible. Even if the patient has no clue about breast cancer at the start, by the time treatments begin a patient is taught more about the condition than ever thought possible.

Fortunately, information and guidelines about breast cancer and different options for unique cases are readily available via the Internet and books. I found out breast cancer is so case specific that even one female may have two different types of breast cancer in her breast(s). A multitude of information is available online. Moreover, the website for the American Cancer Society serves as an informative resource. There are many other available websites, too.

For the most part, Tom and I lived in the hospital for more than two weeks after the biopsy. It took that long to carry out all the required tests before my surgery, a lengthy list of pre-operative procedures. Every day spent in the hospital exhausted me; but they had to check me out from head to toe before they would send me into an operating room. A good hospital *should* thoroughly examine a patient diagnosed with cancer for the purpose of ruling-out any other possible area affected by the disease. By saying that I mean, the doctors needed to consider the metastatic spread of cancerous cells to other body tissue via the blood stream or lymphatic flow and drainage.

It took about three weeks since the day I returned to Dallas to finally complete all of those tests. A follow-up appointment with my doctor was scheduled, and I was looking forward to meeting with her again. Mentally prepared for my operation, I knew I was in reliable hands. Once I trusted my doctors, I was no longer afraid, as much. Finding a doctor who I was comfortable and able to bond with was a miracle to me. In the rigid circumstances of dealing with cancer, it was natural to be worried. Anyone with a serious problem like mine would be worried. Trusting and having faith in the doctor and nursing staff made a surprisingly great difference.

Before I made my final decision about choosing a surgeon or hospital, I spent hours and hours gathering reliable sources of information regarding my treatment plan. Initially, the computer and Internet were my two main resources, until I further explored books at the bookstores. I spoke with cancer survivors who were thoroughly supportive and encouraging. Also, I conducted interviews with doctors and other medical professionals, some friends of mine in the medical field – all wonderful advisors who took a special interest in my case.

"This is the only body I am going to have, for goodness sakes. I have to be sure I received the best possible treatment available to me."

In my endless investigation about making a right decision for my treatment plan, I learned one of the most important parts of my treatment was choosing a top-notch surgeon experienced and specialized. Searching for a hospital affiliated with medical universities or a research-oriented hospital funded by the government could serve well, if affording a private hospital exceeds a patient's budget. Whether a patient is insured by a private sector or needs to employ the programs of a county hospital, one element that applies equally to both avenues is the selection of the right doctor. I made sure I completed my homework industriously.

Given my un-insured situation, I did not have the luxury of choosing any hospital I wanted. I calculated the total cost for my diagnostic tests, surgery, chemo, and radiation therapy to a sum of over one hundred thousand dollars, not to mention any fees associated with follow up visits to the hospital. Because Tom was taking care of me through my recovery, and neither of us worked, we were unable to earn an income. There was no way Tom and I could afford to pay this out of our bank account. Our friends offered loans to us, and Tom considered selling our home to afford paying our bills.

Luckily, I was assigned to a breast specialist surgeon who I trusted. She was working in that county hospital where I positioned myself to be treated. A hospital or clinic could have the highest quality of equipments, but what matters most is if the specialists working there know how to use it.

In many ways, dealing with the hospital facility where I was treated was still a challenging experience; however the one area I was completely satisfied with was my team of medical oncologists. I was lucky because I did not have a choice in the selection of a certain team of surgeons.

The day before my surgery, I went shopping with my husband and since shopping is my favorite thing to do, I decided to keep my mind busy with something I enjoyed. I looked for P.J.'s with soft fabric and an opening in the front to be more comfortable for changing. I found and purchased myself apple-green colored pajamas. I also prepared and ironed two other sets of P.J.'s that I already owned for wearing during my return home from the hospital. I just wanted to look my best.

The night before my surgery, I made a nice hot bath with lavender oils, lit scented candles around the bathtub and turned on soft music.

Sounds pretty juicy, doesn't it?

Well, as another aside, that is why I am writing this book. I am a believer of mind power. I could have sat down in a puddle of stress about what would happen to me in the days ahead and end up with a restless night without sleep. Instead I made a choice to control my environment and set a tone of relaxation.

While in the bathtub, I closed my eyes and imagined my body clear and free of cancer, imagining an entirely healthy body. From above, outside of myself, I looked down to the tub and saw my healthy body soaking in white rose petals with the most pleasant fragrance I have ever smelled floating through the air. It brought a soothing smile to my face.

Tom came to the bathroom door, opening it just enough to peek in to check on me. Since my diagnosis, he followed me like my shadow. I knew he was a nervous wreck and merely putting on a calm front.

"You are a remarkable women who is dealing with this situation in such a way that seems more like a novel than reality," he said, as he checked up on me. "You give me strength and hope. You teach me something new every day by your actions and clear mind." Opening the door fully, he came in and walked to sit at the edge of the tub watching over me like an angel. He went on to suggest, "You could help so many women dealing with the same problems you have by starting a workshop or something. You could share with others the techniques you use to prepare yourself, and maybe later on how you travel the road of recovery." He grabbed my hand and said lovingly, "You are my inspiration each day."

"The night after I found out of my diagnosis, I started writing a diary." I revealed, "Writing is helping me relax and I am pouring my feelings out onto paper and freeing myself. It's how I am able to talk about my fears, my hopes and my dreams." I thought it might end up as a heartwarming little book, but one never knows.

The night before my surgery, part of the pre-op was to fast, without eating or drinking from midnight onward. I had a light dinner at eight o'clock and had my last glass of water for the day at eleven. Because I was scheduled for surgery at seven thirty in the morning, I was supposed to go to bed earlier. But even after my soothing bath, I was just not ready to go to bed yet.

Heather called me that night to say, "Vida, you are in my heart and prayers and I will be with you."

I walked around the house and worked on odds and ends to busy myself and further plan for the next day, then eventually went to bed to sleep.

5
Stage Two

Four-thirty the next morning I awoke. Everything needed was already in place, so all I had left to do was brush my teeth and dress. No makeup, no nail polish, and no lotions – I guess I could deal with that for a little while.

At four forty-five, there was a knock at my front door. A dear family friend came to our house insisting on coming to the hospital with us.

How could I ever repay the amount of love and care I received from people?

As the start-time for surgery neared, my heart and soul remained open to receiving and accepting all the love and prayers being sent in my direction. I had confidence I would turn out just fine. I felt love and devotion from everyone through their encouraging messages and prayers.

The day of my surgery, Tom, Shawn, my dear family friend and I arrived at the hospital at six o'clock in the morning. I remember, the room was as cold as I expected, and the nurse covered me with a blanket. I cracked jokes with my family, keeping the tone light. I don't know what Shawn found attractive about his mom lying in a hospital bed, but he snapped pictures of me with his cell phone.

After one hour of waiting in the room with my family, a man wearing a black gown and a bright smile on his face stepped in.

"I am from the hospital chapel." He said kindly, "Do you wish to receive a prayer before you go for your surgery?" He also asked if I had any specific requests.

"Yes, please. Will you pray and ask God to bless each and every one of the people on my surgical team?" I asked. "Will you also pray for my peace?" We all fell into a focused prayer, as he led us.

Breaking the chill of the room with his silly sense of humor, my husband asked, "I would like an omelet and croissant for breakfast, too." The priest, along with the rest of us, broke into boisterous laughter; and as he was leaving the room, he promised to grant my husband's wishes.

The nurse, anesthesiologist, and resident surgeon walked in to explain the procedures of the surgery – all of them extremely nice and caring. The nurse brought a form of consent needing a signature from me, the patient.

Although a formality and requirement for surgery, the contents of the consent form made me a bit uncomfortable. The nurse read aloud the two pages I was agreeing to with my signature.

"As the patient, you should be aware of the following risk factors during your operation: there is a risk of infection at the site of operation. There is a risk of clot formation that has potential to cause cardiac arrest. In the event of complications due to the use of anesthesia, the patient may not wake up. There is a chance of death due to excessive bleeding."

Wow, quite a contrast from the last visitor in the room: the priest wishing me well and offering blessings. I thought to myself, so much for a patient to agree to right before an operation. Perhaps starting with the consent, and then following with a blessing would have left me more at ease. The consent form caused bundles of stress in the last minute. One would think the moments just before surgery should be filled with hope, reassurance and faith, securing confidence in the events about to occur.

I joked as I signed the from, "I changed my mind and will not be going in for the breast operation."

"I'm sorry, I'm just doing my job." She apologized, understanding the irony.

I managed to successfully handle this last heavy episode of my pre-operative obligations. My husband kissed me, my son kissed me, the nurse wheeled my bed over the threshold out the door, and I left with a smile on my face. As I directed my attention back to Tom and Shawn, I said in my best Arnold Schwarzenegger voice, "I'll be back!"

My operation took about one and half hours. The next thing I knew, the nurse was calling my name.

"Vida, wake up. It's all over."

I could not hear her voice clearly. Amazingly, time passed so quickly. I opened my eyes and was relieved by the realization that I did it! I was out of the operating room. Completely drowsy, I could barely keep my eyes opened.

The nurse said, "You are in the recovery room. Everything is fine."

For a few moments I wondered, "What have they done to my breast? Was it still on my body, still intact?" A warm blanket wrapped my entire body like a cocoon, including my head. I felt cozy. Again my own confirming thoughts echoed in my mind as if I needed more reassurance. "The tumor is out of my body; I made it out of the operating room. Safety!" Then, I fell into a deep slumber.

Some hours later, the nurse began escorting me and the bed back to my own room, an I.V. pumping fluids into my system attached to the post at the head of the bed. Half awake, I began seeing and hearing more clearly. Relief swept through me, as I became more cognitive. As the nurses wheeled my bed through the hallways of the hospital, I saw all of my family waiting near my room, eagerly waving to me. With a weak smile on my face, I waved back and made a victory sign with my fingers pointing to the sky. My husband followed us into the room.

"The surgeon said she was pleased with your operation. She will be stopping by to check on you." Tom informed me as he gently reached for my hand.

I thought to myself in amazement, "How could I have gone through cutting, sawing and come out without feeling the slightest bit of pain?" I was entirely amazed by the power of advanced medicine.

We should all be thankful for science and modern technology enabling the teams of medical professionals to perform miracles of wonder. Grants contributing to advanced research in medicine are helping many women like me to have a chance of living beyond cancer. We are able to carry on with the mission of survival. Scientists are doing a remarkable job in searching for optimal cures. All women should be taking part in the fight against breast cancer through awareness, by becoming educated about prevention and healthier life styles; all women: mothers, sisters, daughters, girl friends. There is never failure with unity, especially when seasoned with love and passion to save lives.

I was extremely dehydrated, and would have given just about anything for a sip of cool water.

When I requested a cold beverage, the recovery nurse said, "You have to wait just a little longer before you may drink water." She continued telling me I would need to slowly intake fluids to allow for my stomach's tolerance to adapt.

Post-operative reactions vary greatly from person to person. I did not experience nausea or vomiting, however the throbbing of my head made it feel like a balloon being continually inflated.

As soon as I was able to drink, the recovery nurse brought me a small glass of water, making me very happy. I slept most of that day in the hospital, with Tom at my side.

Late in the evening I was released to go home. I was very happy to know I could sleep in my own bed with the comfort of being in my own house.

Currently, most hospitals release patients the same or the next day after a surgery. I am not sure if it is a good idea to send a patient home the same day as a partial mastectomy or lumpectomy.

The doctors told me to drink plenty of water to help clear my system of the medication induced for tracing parts of my anatomy during the surgery.

I do not remember much of that night after we arrived home. In a bit of a daze, I just wanted to sleep. I opened my eyes only to drink water. Something I do remember though, was waking up frequently to use the bathroom. I had been drinking so much water to quench my thirst. I remember when I used the bathroom for the first time back at my house. I saw my urine was cobalt blue in color – the same color as the sanitizing tablet we put in the toilet bowl.

"Tom!" I called out. "Did you put a tablet in our toilet?" I was surprised because he had never cleaned a bathroom in his life.

"No, why?" He asked.

"Because my pee is blue!"

"Oh," he laughed. "I forgot to warn you that your doctor said to check for a blue pee, from the dye they injected into your breast." He explained how the injection dyed the sentinel lymph node for the doctor to trace during my surgery.

A few days before my surgery, I had been sent for a sentinel lymph node graph at the breast-imaging center in the county hospital. At that time, the radiologist made an injection of a tiny amount of radioactive substance into my left breast. Following the injection, the radiologist took a computerized image, marked the location of the sentinel lymph node with a black marker and had sent me home. The sentinel lymph node (also referred to as 'the gate keeper') was where the surgeon made an incision about two inches long near my armpit, in order to take a tissue sample to send to the lab. After the surgery I was told there were not any cancerous cells found in the sentinel lymph node and so no lymph nodes were removed during my surgery.

The initial findings on the ultrasound revealed the tumor to be 1.2 centimeters small and in the eight o'clock position. This finding classified my cancer to be in the Stage One category. The initial treatment plan started with a six or seven week healing process for the breast tissue, then six weeks of radiation therapy. After the tumor was removed and sent to the pathology lab, the pathologist reported the actual size of my tumor was 3.5 centimeters large, increasing my classification from a Stage One to a Stage Two. The change in my classification also changed my treatment plan. Because the size of the tumor was 3.5 centimeters in size, the doctors recommended chemotherapy, followed by radiation therapy.

My first reaction was "Oh no! Chemo?"

But my doctor said, "It is your decision whether or not you want to do a combination of chemo and radiation therapy, or just radiation therapy." She also said, "If I was in your position with a 3.5 centimeter tumor, I would definitely choose to do chemotherapy. Although the lymph nodes were not involved, the size of your tumor is a concern. You do not want to take any chances for a possible systemic spread of the cancer."

Believe me when I say it was not easy to decide my own treatment. There were so many issues involved, especially considering and weighing out all of the pros and cons. The positive aspect of chemo is that it obviously kills cancerous cells. While the negative aspect of chemo is that it weakens the immune system, in addition to a long list of other side effects such as, organ failure. I thought back to all the articles I read during the research I conducted to educate myself at the beginning of this lengthy process. I scrolled through hundreds of reputable and resourceful websites to educate myself about each possible treatment for breast cancer.

The type of cancer I was diagnosed with was estrogen positive. As a result of the pathology lab studies conducted, the pathologists concluded that estrogens would trigger and promote the growth of cancer cells in my body, meaning I needed to avoid estrogens of any kind. The doctors then created a treatment plan for me based on all of the specific findings from my lab work, including the results from the pathology lab.

I also learned, as I mentioned earlier, to stay away from all soy products. I lived with soy products as part of my diet for as long as I could remember: from soymilk to tofu, and on and on.

I thought, "How in the hell would I know that my estrogen level was high? My gynecologist never told me anything about estrogens. I thought soy was a cancer-fighting agent; and the more soy in my diet, the better my health would be. I did not know I was putting poison into my precious body."

As they say, "Wake up and smell the roses."

I was awakened; I woke up and smelled the soy.

The moral of the soy sob story is please check with your gynecologist to see whether your estrogen and progesterone levels are within normal ranges.

Not only did I stop using soy, I read all the labels of foods and products I planned to consume or bring near my body, making sure they did not contain soy as an ingredient. I paid close attention to, for instance, breakfast cereals, nutrition bars, even shampoos, conditions and soaps. I was surprised when I found soy oil as an ingredient in sore throat lozenges. My question became how could I clear all the soy from my body's delicate system? The answer: I could not. Without a strict detoxification program, my body's natural cleansing process would have to run its course.

Patients are mostly left with the responsibility of dredging up facts about miracle foods that can assist with cleansing the body. For more information about natural medicine, I logged onto www.IamMD.com. I also read research at the Johns Hopkins website regarding nutrition in respect to assisting with treating breast cancer; they offer a newsletter with the latest research – just one of many great resources.

It is believed that Cancer feeds on sugars, and fat. Cancer cells find the oxygen-deprived tissue in the body where they seek to take over, reside and multiply. Cancer cells are unable to sustain their life in an oxygen-rich environment. Cancer can be managed with properly balanced nutrition. Every minute in a day the body's immune system kills-off cancer cells, working to create a homeostatic balance. As long as the human body remains in balance, the cancer cells will not be able to proliferate or multiply. A Nobel Prize was awarded to the German biochemist, Otto Warburg, for his discoveries of the metabolism of cancer cells. Warburg's studies concluded, "Cancer has only one prime cause. It is the replacement of normal oxygen respiration of the body's cells by an anaerobic (i.e., oxygen-deficient) cell respiration." Meaning, carcinogens thrive when oxygen is not present in the body. His own research made him fearful of processed foods.

Cancer stinks!

Do not fall prey as an uninformed victim. Please take charge for your own life, make informed decisions, read research and know about your disease and the treatment options; consult professionals versed in treatments to prevent and treat cancer. Learn the do's and do not's. Nobody cares about you nor can care for you more than yourself. Do you really want to fight cancer? Decide, then move on and be proactive with healing. It will help you. I speak from personal experience and based a book upon my experience. I want to stand on the soapbox to share what I did not previously know, and teach other women to avoid the mistakes I made.

Whether a movie star, a housewife, or even the wife of the President of the United States, we are all equal. When a cancer patient, it does not matter one small bit who you are: you are sick, a most equaling situation. An ordinary woman, like myself with breast cancer: sick.

As a matter of fact, I read a book written by Fran Drescher, commonly know as 'Nanny,' entitled *Cancer Schmancer*. She talks about how her uterine cancer was misdiagnosed as a pre-menopausal condition and how she was juggled from one doctor to another; and by the time the cancer in her uterus was found, two years had elapsed; how frightening. Sometimes it is better to be nobody than to be mistreated or misjudged. In her book, she was urging women to pursue second opinions, even third opinions. What I am trying to say is find all the help available, and stop searching only when all questions have been answered.

I am trying to include every little detail about my experience over the course of my diagnosis, treatment, and recovery. I want to touch on every point that might be helpful for women who deal with breast cancer, their own or that of a loved one.

I became deeply frightened with the decision of having to choose chemo or not. I have always been scared of chemotherapy because it has many dangerous affects on the body. Chemotherapy could be perceived as a brutal attack to all of the rapidly dividing cells in the body, such as the hair follicles and the cells of the body's immune system. There is so much controversy surrounding chemotherapy and its use with cancer patients. The long list of side effects associated with chemotherapy includes: tiredness and fatigue, nausea and vomiting, numbness and tingling, diarrhea and/or constipation, hair loss, mouth sores, skin irritations, loss of appetite, change in taste, anxiety, difficulty sleeping, infertility, cognitive impairment, liver damage, kidney damage, an increase in susceptibility to infections, lowered blood pressure due to a decrease in red blood cells, white blood cells and blood platelets.

The extent of side effects a patient could experience depends upon the particular type of chemo administered, the drug dosage, and the body's reactions to it. Chemotherapy has been used to kill off tumor cells, however, in the process also kills many of the naturally growing cells in the body. The main idea is to attempt to kill off as many of the cancerous cells as possible, and hope that when the treatment is through there are still enough healthy cells in the body to carry on life.

I was scared of it, just like kids are scared of monsters.

I did not want to lose my hair or be bald. I did not want to feel sicker than I already felt. I did not want poison entering my body. I did not want to throw up! I had witnessed people going through chemotherapy and I did not want to be one of them.

Not too long ago I lost a good friend to breast cancer. I remember talking with her when she complained about the side effects she was experiencing as a result of her chemotherapy treatment. In the late stages of her treatment, the doctors asked her to under-go a second term of chemo and she refused.

I remember my trip to Ohio to spend a week with her, devastated to hear the news about her breast cancer. I was begging her to seek proper treatment.

It was three days after her surgery when I arrived to Ohio. Her husband picked me up from the airport. He and I talked during the drive until we arrived at their house.

"The doctors said the size of her tumor was about the size of a tennis ball!" Her husband reported.

"How did that happen?" I asked, shocked at the thought of a tennis ball sized tumor growing inside the body of my dear friend.

"It is an aggressive type of cancer that the doctors say grew between the period of her previous mammogram and her most recent one."

When we arrived to her house, she was so happy to see me and looked adorable without hair. Her head looked like a little pumpkin, perfectly round. Her eyebrows and eyelashes had fallen out, too. She had been receiving chemotherapy even prior to her mastectomy to reduce the size of the tumor and a few months after surgery, had more chemotherapy. There was a small clear bag attached at the incision site of the mastectomy where I could see the fluid drainage leaking out into the bag. She had to measure the amount of fluid daily.

Strong and happy to still be alive, she said, "I will survive this because I want to see my little girl grow up; I want to see her as a beautiful bride one day."

In those few days, I helped her in everyway I could think of: drawing baths for her, making fresh-squeezed vegetable and fruit juices each day, preparing healthy meals. I gave her all I could offer.

She promised, "I'm going to eat healthy from now on, and stay active!"

She wore size sixteen and I worried that her bad eating habits and lack of exercise could be negative contributing factors to her treatment. She agreed with me, and for six months was committed to walking every day and eating as healthy as she could possibly eat. She lost so much weight, and was thereafter a size twelve. My friend changed her lifestyle for a while, but fell back into her old habit of eating fatty foods and sugars. I remember cleaning out her refrigerator while staying with her. There were loads of pies, macaroni and cheese, cold cuts, and cookies just to mention some of what I found.

Some of her well-intentioned friends delivered ready-made fast foods, thinking they were helping her to reduce the effort required for preparing her own meals.

When I was living overseas, I used to call her to check in. She admitted that due to her busy lifestyle she did not have time to go for walks anymore. Nor did she have time to prepare special meals for her to sustain healthy eating.

"The cancer will come back if you don't take care of yourself," I told her. Again, she agreed with me and promised to be more active and eat healthier.

In less than two years cancer paid her another visit. Of course, she was devastated. The cancer metastasized, spreading all over my poor friends' body. I could not believe it. I can still remember our conversation about how I warned her about lifestyle habits, and told her ways to amend her diet and exercise routine. Perhaps she may have lived a little longer if she would have take better care of herself. At this late stage in her cancer treatment, she was refusing to finish the chemotherapy.

"I can not take it anymore! CANCER SUCKS!" She said. This visit from cancer was a fatal one.

At that time, I did not realize that two years after her deah I would be a cancer victim myself and have to ask for her help from up in heaven, requesting her soul's healing energy to shine down upon me.

Do I want to make a wrong decision because of moments of frustration? Absolutely not.

From the moment I was diagnosed with cancer, chemo was my worst nightmare; that was what I dreaded more than the surgery. Could I overcome my fear of?

6
Inner Self: Soul

I went to my meditation spot and sat down quietly, praying to God to help me regain my mental strength. I reminded myself how important it was to believe in myself.

"Stop getting so emotional." I coached myself, "It happens when you are tired and ill, you can lose control and become frustrated." I knew it was okay for me to lose control every now and then, but only if I had the ability to pull back on the reigns, bringing my frustration to a halt.

Each of my meditation sessions elevated my confidence and energy levels. My meditative inward glances were the fuel for my uplifted and positive frame of mind. Also, Tom was my angel; his true love and care pulled me through many of my struggles. He supported me, fed me and continually encouraged me.

A month after my surgery, while my breast tissue was still in a healing phase, Tom and I traveled to California for a wedding. I had my hair professionally highlighted, and figured a trip to California would pump-me-up before I started my treatment with chemo and radiation therapy. Our week in California turned out to be the most fun trip ever. Being surrounded by family and friends, as well as being witness to the lovely wedding ceremony was absolutely the most wonderful medicine to heal my soul. The icing on the cake was Shawn joining us at the wedding. I was so happy to have it all. I returned back home with a pocket full of fun memories.

The day after our return, I had an appointment with my medical oncologist to discus my treatment plan. I started questioning my doctor about my options.

"Is there a way for me to skip the chemotherapy?" I hoped. She suggested doing a test called an Oncotype Test, a quantitative assessment of the likelihood of disease reoccurrence. The test score would reveal the level of risk involved for remission or reoccurrence.

"Not a bad test to try," I thought.

Because the test could not be performed in the hospital and was an elective procedure, it turned out to be a little pricey. Since the test was performed at my request and not a part of my treatment plan, I was responsible for paying the bill.

But hey, I've got one life to live. I'm worth it.

The pathology lab had the sample of my breast tissues saved in the lab from my previous biopsy. The tissue needed to be sent out of the hospital to a lab specialist to perform the Oncotype Test. The results of the test would dictate the course of my treatment. If the score was low enough, chemotherapy would not be recommended.

After two long weeks of waiting, the score finally came back. The medical oncologist went through the test results with me, teaching me how to evaluate the reoccurrence score.

"There are three categories of results: low risk, inter-mediate risk, and high risk."

If my score fell into the low risk category, I would have been off the hook and would not need chemotherapy. However, if my reoccurrence score landed in the category of medium to high risk, I would without a doubt be recom-mended to go through chemotherapy.

"Your score is in between the categories of low and in-termediate risk." She said.

There I was on the score chart swinging right in the middle between low and intermediate risk, leaning slightly closer to the low risk as compared to intermediate.

My oncologist said, "If I was wearing your shoes, I would do the chemotherapy to gain peace of mind."

I did not argue about the matter any longer. I had to do what I had to do.

The hospital scheduled me for the first round of chemo-therapy three days after I met with my medical oncologist.

Without exaggeration, I tell you, I was in hell for those three days turning over all of the ideas I had in my mind about chemotherapy. I did not want to go through chemo-therapy. Really, who does? I was so disappointed with life and everything else; I cried an ocean of tears. I didn't know what was happening to me.

I just plain *did not know*.

By the recommendation of the oncologist, I said I would start the chemo.

As the first day for chemotherapy quickly approached, I did not know what to do. On one hand I was doubled over with the stress of being so scared about chemo, and on the other hand I wanted to reduce the risks of a possible remission. I hid my fearful emotions from the man I love so much, not wanting him to be burdened by my chemo dilemma.

I was getting tired of my own weakness and realized having anxiety about my treatment was not going to work for me.

In the early morning before the first treatment of che-motherapy, I awoke around three. I sat up, and my mind immediately flooded-over with the nervousness of going to the hospital to be subjected to chemotherapy.

"How can I stop chemotherapy from happening... somehow. But how?" My thoughts tossed and turned. "I need rest. Tomorrow is going to be a very long day at the hospital." My mind ran around skipping in angst. Sleep had already abandoned my exhausted eyes. Tired of my own weakness, I realized being internally divided was not going to hinder my ability to heal. After a few minutes of tossing thoughts around, I sat up on my bed and started talking to myself out loud.

"If I don't do something about this fear of chemotherapy, not only am I going to be miserable for the next few months, but my body may reject the medicine. The results could be a total disaster." I continued talking to myself like a mad woman.

"Okay, here is the total scenario." I raised my right hand, "Chemo." I barely started to raise my left hand, "Cancer. Right or left; which one am I going to choose: Cancer or Chemo?"

I thought, "Do I let my fear take over and mess up the treatment?"

"I better not!" I told myself, jumping out my bed with an idea. I walked into my bathroom, pulled open the drawer where I kept my hairpins; I grabbed my headband. Then went to the desk to pick up two markers: red and black. I started writing on my headband: "I LOVE CHEMO." (I drew a red heart for love). "CANCER SUCKS!!"

This silly little headband made me smile, changing my entire attitude. I strapped it around my forehead and went back. I was able to go back to sleep for a few more hours.

The headband particularly tickled me when I looked into the mirror the next morning and it was still wrapped around my head. Wearing it gave me amazing strength so I kept it on as I left the house to go for my treatment.

Making my way through the hospital towards the oncology department for my first chemotherapy, everybody was smiling at me, admiring my gutsy pride in wearing that headband. People seemed to love the way I was expressing my feelings about cancer. Boy, I tell you, that headband made my fears go to hell! At least it was a start for some one like me, a step towards accepting my situation.

The first cycle of chemo took about two hours. The registered nurse injected the medicine through a rectangular shaped Mediport, a little device made with special materials used to facilitate the delivery of the chemo medication directly into my blood stream. The Mediport, a soft chamber with a diameter about the size of a nickel, connected to a tiny long tube. I was under local anesthesia as the Mediport was placed under the skin on the healthy side of my chest wall, just a few inches below my clavicle. The tiny tube was inserted inside a large vein in my neck, and was then fixed to the skin by a few stitches.

A week after implanting the Mediport, they started my chemotherapy. The advantage of using the Mediport was that each time I returned for a chemo treatment, I did not have to be poked in the arms or anywhere else for an injection. The chemotherapy drugs were very strong, and had the potential of causing a local irritation at the injection site. For that reason, as well as for patient comfort and ease of treatment some doctors prefer the use of a Mediport.

Each visit, the nurse flushes the Mediport with saline before injecting the chemotherapy medication. Some doctors recommend keeping the Mediport for a year just in case there was a need for another round of chemotherapy. I asked for mine to be removed two months after my radiation therapy was done.

During the chemotherapy, I requested a blanket because the temperature in the room felt freezing cold. Throughout the treatment, I drank water like a fish to keep my body well hydrated. Although I would finish a big bottle of water during each chemotherapy session, I still felt dehydrated.

Drinking plenty of water assisted with cleansing my body. I studied about the possible side effects chemotherapy could have on the kidneys; and drinking plenty of fluids – especially filtered water – aids in the kidney's ability to remove toxic wastes from the blood stream.

Who wants to be healed of breast cancer but have a kidney failure in the process?

My doctor recommended consuming between four and six extra glasses of water than I normally drank. Since ingesting plenty of water was already a part of my daily routine, I increased my liquid intake from eight glasses a day to about twelve or fourteen. I was perfectly okay with the excess water, though it made for more frequent visits to the ladies room.

I finished the first cycle of my chemotherapy and walked out of the hospital with my husband by my side. One cycle done and seven more to go.

When we arrived home, I had soup for lunch and took a long nap. Tom took charge of my food preparation to make sure I ate healthy meals. Taking caution to avoid cross contamination, he paid particularly close attention to keeping the kitchen unsoiled, clean and tidy. Even though Tom disliked washing dirty dishes, during my treatments he washed the dishes and cleaned the entire kitchen with pleasure. He prepared foods flavored with love and the aroma of his lentil soup sure woke up my poor appetite. Over time, our friends that stopped by to check up on me during their lunch breaks became Tom's regular lunch costumers. After eating his delicious lentil soup, my body seemed to be directing me to rest. The day after chemotherapy, I was extremely tired and stayed in bed pretty much all day long feeling nauseated. Luckily I did not throw-up, and to me that was a blessing.

The few days following the chemotherapy, I ate very small portions of cooked meals, but still did not have much of an appetite. I was told to avoid eating raw fish, raw vegetables and fruits. I only consumed fruits with thick skin, because chemotherapy weakens the immune system. By ridding my diet of raw foods, the possibility of becoming sick would be lowered. Basically, I avoided germs and bacteria that could potentially enter into my digestive or respiratory systems. I ate only steamed or cooked vegetables and avoided salads. Tom did not buy any pre-cut vegetables. He thoroughly washed and cut all of the produces in our own kitchen.

The fruits I ate during the treatment consisted of melons, bananas, pineapples and mangos. Other fruits like apples and pears or peaches were all baked in the oven or steamed. Extreme precaution was taken especially during my chemotherapy treatment. All of the foods we purchased were organic. I was already paying an enormous price for fighting the invader, and to kick it out of my system required proper nutrition to boost the function of my immune system. I wanted to eat the highest quality foods.

During the period of my chemotherapy treatments, I avoided going to public places, especially on weekends and busy hours. By saying that, I did not isolated myself, by any means. But if I wanted to shop, I chose the hours when the stores were least crowded.

In addition, when our family and friends came over to our house, we made sure they were not carrying a cold or flu along for their visit. We asked visitors to come a few days after my chemotherapy, when I was a little stronger and not quite as tired as the day of or the days just after being treated. We requested only two or a maximum of three visitors per day. I took all safeguards.

Whenever we planned to go to a restaurant, which was seldom, we only selected places where we felt comfortable as well as places we felt provided a sanitary environment. Frequently ordering *off* the menu, I requested dishes to be specially cooked and tailored for me: essentially ordering low in fat, low in salt, fully cooked meals. Every chef we encountered was willing to cater to my dietary needs.

During my entire cancer treatment, I stayed away from nightshade growing produces like potatoes, mushrooms, and eggplant. As part of a macrobiotic cooking method, my husband prepared and cooked organic foods for us. To learn more about macrobiotic cooking, I logged-on to www.christophercenter.org/cooking.html.

Refined carbohydrates such as pastas, rices and refined sugars were all eliminated from my diet as well. It's believed that sugar and fat feed cancer cells, so I kept them away from me during chemo and continued avoiding them long after my treatment ended. I did eat some sweets occasionally though. Since I am a chocolate lover, I found organic and dark chocolates to treat myself often enough.

My designed diet was based on my own research dis-coveries, and personally it worked for me. A diet for anyone else should be tailored to meet one's own individual needs. Consult a doctor or a nutritionist and be sure to eat a balanced diet during and after cancer treatments. Since we are all different, one person's diet may not work for everyone. Please consult with a professional, better yet conduct your own research and become actively involved with learning about nutrition and its benefits.

During my chemotherapy treatment I did not drink green tea because it contains properties that had potential to interfere with my treatments. Everything I purchased had to be free of soy products, even body lotions. I read labels carefully checking all ingredients. My grocery shopping was fairly time consuming, however I was the leader of my own crusade in this war against breast cancer. Never underestimate the enemy. A healthy food intake was the first line of my defense on the home front. Fresh squeezed vegetables and fruits were like juices of life, my ammunition.

On the fifth day of my first chemotherapy cycle, I started taking short walks and asked my husband to be my escort and accompany me. He came for walks with me the first two days; then he quit. He was the iron chef of the kitchen, but not so interested in being the iron-man of the outdoors. We all have different points of interest. Tom is a phenomenal chef, and as long as he does not have to go for walks, he is willing to help me.

One morning when I was walking along the sidewalk in my neighborhood, my next-door neighbor stopped me and started chatting.

"Where have you been over the past two months?" She asked.

When I told her what happened to me, she was surprised how calmly I spoke of my experiences.

"You are such a great example for other women" she said. She told me the story of her sister in-law, who was diagnosed with breast cancer. "Can I have her contact you for some advice?"

"It is my pleasure," I told her. "If I can be of any help, I would love to speak with her."

The next day I went for my regular walk and about thirty minutes later, returned home sweaty and hungry. After taking a cool shower, I ate a delicious breakfast. Tom and I cleaned up the kitchen together, and I was feeling great. The two of us decided to go out shopping, one of my favorite pass-times.

Around one o'clock in the afternoon, I felt an unusual pain on my side near my kidneys traveling down into my low back. The pain felt extremely sharp like an electric shock, but didn't last very long, so I tried to ignore it. Five minutes later, the pain returned more severely than the first time, and was pulsating. In my opinion, nothing is more annoying than a mystery pain, not knowing where it was coming from or why it occurred. I learned to be prepared for uninvited pain.

Looking back, I know I experienced random pains every now and again as a result of the chemotherapy. When my cycle of chemo ended, so did the mysterious pains.

7
Vibrant Connection

The second week after my first chemo, I realized I was losing hair.

"Why is my hair falling out so fast; what is the rush?" I thought. "And only in the second week of treatment."

In the beginning, my hair was about shoulder length and very full. During my showers, I came to the shocking realization that a woman's hair is her confidant. My hair matted the showers floor, covering and clogging the drain. I no longer looked forward to showering. I did not deserve that shit!

Oh, the fatigue, lack of appetite, upset stomach, hair loss, and random pains all became too much for me to handle, attacking me all at once like an invasion on my soul. I felt like a little girl and as reliant as a baby needing her mother.

"Why do I feel so vulnerable? How could I not be venerable? I am a woman. I am a human, hurting so deeply. No matter what anyone says to offer a dose of comfort, I am facing this physical and emotional terror on my own."

Then, one morning as I was showering, my hair became tangled in knots even after I used a large handful of conditioner. I did not know what to do with my hair. It was very unusual to me because I never before in my life had a tangled hair. It was a fuzz ball, though. My arms became exhausted from just rinsing my hair, trying to untangle the knots. I pulled out as much of the dead hair as I could. I don't know how long I was crying under the showers' rain; all I remember was the hot water turned cold before I could finish. I stepped out of the cold shower and looked at myself in the mirror. I looked like a woman wearing a Halloween costume, a baldheaded clown with only strings of hair hanging down.

"Vida?" I heard my husband calling my name, and I ran into my closet to hide myself.

"He already has enough to handle," I thought.

After looking in the bedroom, he found me in the closet and we held each other crying.

Finally, when I stopped crying, which took a good long while, I asked Tom to shave my head.

For the past fifteen years I have been his personal barber and this was pay back time! I could not believe in my wildest dreams the day would come for me to ask him to shave my head. He really tried to cheer me up by saying how cute I looked with my baldhead.

In later stages of my recovery, I looked back thinking my vulnerable bald look was somewhat sexy. But at the time it was a slap in the face.

It screamed: *You Have Cancer!*

It made it impossible to forget the disease had invaded my life.

So, there I was bald, everything creeping on my nerves, having to deal with one more dilemma. I should have cut my hair short before any of it began falling out. But I thought I had plenty of time to enjoy my hair with its brand new highlights put in before my chemo for the wedding we attended in California. At first, my hair was hardly shedding and I did not sense any urgency to cut it so soon. Chemotherapy affects people in different ways. My hair loss started long before I anticipated and long before I was ready.

One of my girlfriends surprised me when she said she was going to shave *her* head so I didn't have to be alone. I knew she meant it and her gesture truly touched my heart. My husband also decided he would shave his head. I knew I had to seriously stop him, because Tom is a fast acting kind of man. I love his hair thick, grayish in color with the most beautiful curls, manly of course. The last thing I wished to see around the house was another bald head.

Losing my hair did not stop me from my outdoor activities. I continued walking wearing a hat. I started a little earlier than I used to in order to avoid unwanted attention from curious neighbors. But it didn't take long for them to find out about my cancer, probably faster than my gynecologist overseas! At any rate, the neighbors were all very supportive. I was surprised when every single woman in my neighborhood had a story to tell of one friend or another, or even members of their family who dealt with breast cancer.

The woman who lived right next-door, a very sweet and funny lady, told me, "Just two weeks ago my aunt *and* my aunt's best friend were *both* diagnosed with breast cancer."

I was furious.

What is wrong in our country? Is cancer epidemic? Is there something wrong with our bras? What is in our food, our water, our air? Something is definitely wrong. I hope all the funds going towards breast cancer research are well spent, not solely dedicated to finding a cure but more importantly the cause.

Over the telephone, Heather told me a story about a woman she knew who was diagnosed with breast cancer. Shortly after the woman realized her own condition, she learned that two of her closest friends were diagnosed with breast cancer also. They were raised and grew up in the same town. Coincidence?

These three women decided to conduct a search, and sure enough discovered seven other women in their hometown around their same age were also diagnosed with various types of cancer.

When I heard their tale, I again had the same compelling questions: What is going on? Is cancer epidemic? Is something in our food, our clothes, our water, our environment causing cancer? Where the hell is it coming from and who has the answers to my futile questions?

You may frequently hear of the survival rate, but do you ever see a decline of the rate of occurrence of breast cancer? Just about everyone I talk to has a family member or knows someone diagnosed with cancer. This is not-at-all a slight matter. It's not the damn flu! Cancer is a disease that destroys lives, a terrible disease that puts people through hell until it either kills them or they are able to prevail over its viciousness. Even those who recover know the need is ever present to continually be on alert for its remission. New studies show cancer can strike again ten to fifteen years even after a full recovery. Cancer is a nasty disease that changes people's lives, their priorities, and their direction. This disease scars people's lives.

We must ask who or what is responsible for all of these sorrows? Do we deserve this? Does anybody deserve this?

I didn't think so.

I have learned not to hold any of my feelings inside any more. The reason I opened up to talking about my frustrations, my disappointments, as well as my Kodak moments is for a release from them. Instead of holding everything inside, women should let go of stress; it is poisonous. I paid an enormous price when I let it constrain me. Stress ignited my hormones and my imbalanced condition and put me through so much pain and suffering I didn't want any other woman to have to experience.

I am going to share the story of a woman who truly touched my life with her wisdom. Back in 1987, when Tom and I lived in Charlotte, North Carolina, our house was in a country setting. I remember the charming characteristics of the town, the early-style American homes residing on Queen Street. Very large, old trees with wide spreading branches entangled over the pavement created a green tunnel above the street. For the first few months of living in Charlotte, my husband and I had picnics every weekend to enjoy our quaint picturesque natural surroundings, very different from Texas.

Around the corner from the farm road leading to our house, Tom and I noticed a small wooden sign hung on a post reading: 'Antiques.' We could not really see the shop. Every time we drove by, we were overcome with curiosity and had to find out if it was really an antique shop. One day We slowly drove under the branches at the entrance to the hidden drive, wondering if someone might appear with a shotgun. Because it was private property, we drove slowly and carefully into the driveway looking for people or watchdogs. Just inside the entrance from the road, trees all around, and no indication for alarm, we stayed in the car looking all around us waiting a minute, but no one showed up. It was very peaceful and quiet, and there was a large house down at the end of the driveway.

As soon as we decided to make a U-turn to leave, a tall strong woman with short shiny gray hair wearing blue jeans stepped-through the front door of the house. She was in her seventies or so, and had a solid build. Her friendly smile lit up her face.

"How can I help you?" She said, moving closer to our car.

"Is the antique shop open?" I asked through the car window.

"Well no, not really." She said looking up, seeming to reference the back of her mind. "It has been almost ten years since the shop's been open. But let me show you 'round, if you'd like."

We stepped out of our car, and followed her towards a barn across from the main house. Her house was charmingly nestled in the most beautiful landscape with over three acres of land. My attention was drawn by the sound of the softly trickling waterfall pouring over rocks into a little pond with water lilies, home to koi fish. Next to the pond, a small wooden bench was perched under a willow bend tree. In amazement of the scenery of her hidden treasure, I stopped walking for a moment to admire the beauty.

On her main land beside the pecan and fruit trees, it looked as if the flowering roses were part of a professionally landscaped display of nature.

"Come on, let me show you inside the barn where the antique shop used to be. Then I can give you a tour through the house." She said, so inviting and friendly.

Antiques, flowers, pecan trees and a fishpond on gorgeous landscape – I felt like I was in heaven!

"I'm Tom," my husband said, reaching out for an introductory handshake. "And this is my wife Vida."

"My name is Ann," she replied, as she kindly shook both of our hands.

"We are new in town; we live right around the corner." I said, pointing across her land towards the dirt road where we entered.

Scanning her antique stock, we saw just about every knick-knack one could imagine, from old darkened garden tools and pottery, to weathervanes, glass vases, and old jar containers. The barn was set up like a captured memory of her antique shop when it was in business. As she told us about the antiques, she presented herself as a brilliant woman, and very sweet. She reminded me of my grand-mother who passed away, full of wisdom. We walked through the barn like long lost friends.

The woman noticed my gaze focused on the raw fruits lying on the windowsill drying.

"My trees harvest so much food that it almost goes to waste. I make jam preserves with some of the fruits and dry the others to give to family and friends."

I remembered her estate was so beautiful I didn't want to leave. I wanted to stay longer. After we finished the tour of her house and the plush gardens we started to say good-bye. Before we left, she handed me a bag of pecans and a couple of peaches and blackberry preserves.

"Please come back sometime soon." To my surprise, she invited me for another visit. "I certainly do enjoy visitors."

"Yes," I replied eagerly. "I would love to visit again."

I later learned she was actually eighty years old the day I met her. She looked so much younger; I wondered her secret to upholding youthfulness.

"Thank you for taking us in." We waved good-bye as we drove out of her long dirt driveway.

Waving, she yelled out to us, "Hope to see you again soon."

Ann became a very good friend of mine. She told me her life story and how she took care of her husband and his health problems; he was six years younger than her. Also, her mother-in-law was in the hospital.

"I cut flowers from the garden, and bake breads to bring to my mother-in-law to brighten her days." She told me.

That was interesting, an eighty-year-old woman had a *living* mother in law! How old might *she* be? Even at the ripe age of eighty Ann took charge of caring for herself and her family. Ann was very organized and active with swimming three times a week and walking thirty minutes a day. Not to mention she also mowed the lawn and landscaped the lovely gardens throughout her estate.

One day while she pruned her peach tree, I asked her, "How do you do this? Doesn't all the work become exhausting?"

She said to me, "Work is good for you. One must always keep the mind busy and moving productively. It makes me happy. You know what kills people?" She continued, "Stress!"

When she and I had this discussion, I was too young to realize the weight of the precious anecdote she attempted to illustrate for me. Never the less, I have her story filed in my memory. I often think about her and I know she is enjoying taking care of her heavenly gardens.

As Ann said, "Stress is the biggest and most dangerous killer." She was not a doctor or a scientist, but was able to recognize the truth about mind power and motion. She was living proof of a woman with an incandescent mind yielding a healthy body. She lived in an oasis of nature surrounded by all that she loved. Her positive outlook along with her active hobbies made it possible for her to live a long and happy life free from stress.

At the end of each cycle of chemo, my appetite usually increased back to normal and I took advantage of my desire to eat. Tom stirred up delicious meals to fuel my body in the attempt of increasing my strength for the next round of chemotherapy. Only two weeks remained before it was time for me to go back to the hospital for the next chemo treatment. Tom's non-stop effort to keep me energized with healthy food and his undying love kept me going strong.

My blood sample was sent to the lab each time before starting another round of chemotherapy. After about two hours waiting in the treatment room, the results came in and so did the oncologist. She reviewed the blood test findings to rule out any possible kidney or liver damage that may have occurred as a result of the chemotherapy. Blood tests were a snap shot of what was going on inside my body at a given point in time. Almost every time I went for a treatment, most of my day was spent in the hospital.

The original plan of my treatment was eight cycles of chemotherapy, every other week for sixteen weeks. When I went for the second cycle, a new oncologist was placed incharge of my treatment. The new doctor, a very knowledgeable new graduate, was supervised by the original doctor. The county hospital where I received my treatment was associated with a medical university. Each patient's treatment protocol was managed by a group of doctors: interns, staff doctors, resident doctors, as well as the head of the breast oncology department. The head of the department approved all major decisions regarding patient treatments. Each patient had an assigned staff doctor and it was not unusual to see a change of assignment.

My new oncologist was extremely brilliant and well prepared to start her own practice. Since my cancer had not spread into my lymph nodes, and despite its size of 3.5 centimeters, she believed I would be better served with a less aggressive approach to my treatment. She discussed her point of view with the head of the breast oncology department. Their decision to reduce my treatment by three cycles of chemo from the original eight prescribed, as well as to reduce the medication to a less aggressive form was the best news I could have possibly heard. Yes, three less cycles of chemotherapy! In addition, the new oncologist believed with the lowered intensity of the medication I would no longer experience nausea, and would have a better tolerance towards the overall treatment. She really made my day. Inflated with joy and energy, I totally forgot about my hair loss. Less chemotherapy would end my treatment course much sooner than expected, allowing me enough time to prepare for Christmas celebrations.

As soon as I arrived home, I picked up the phone and called all of my friends and son to report the great news. Everyone was so happy for me; they all knew how much I loved the holidays. The new plan made it possible for me to finish the follow-up radiation therapy a whole week before Christmas.

I went back to the hospital three weeks later to receive one of the newly prescribed courses of chemo and everything went well.

That night I had a few people over to the house, and I looked good. With my makeup and a cute little outfit, no one could have possibly thought I had cancer. Actually, my face was very deceiving for someone undergoing chemo. I decided to wear one of the wigs I purchased awhile back. I had several, each with a different style. With the wig, my delicate make up, a healthy diet, and a generally positive outlook on life, I presented as anything except ill. All of my friends teased me a little.

"Are you *sure* you even have cancer?" I took their teasing as a compliment.

During my early morning walks I felt entirely connected with the universe and its healing powers. I was full of love for life. While walking, I carefully observed the neighborhood's landscape. Touching the trunks of each tree I passed by, smelling the fresh fragrance from the flowers, leaves, and newly mowed grasses; I felt the essence of vitality in every little movement. The sky appeared a more translucent blue than ever and the white clouds more vibrant than even Michelangelo's painting at the Sistine Chapel.

Practically talking to nature, telling the flowers of the beauty they possess, I said, "My God, I feel completely connected to your universe unlike ever before." Eyes wide open to appreciate God's gifts, and filled with His unconditional love, I moved in rhythm with His intended song of life.

"Are all of my awakenings because of cancer?"

I realized my emotions could change from happy to sad, from excitement to bored, from feeling great to feeling exhausted; and I learned to nurture myself and not to suppress or hold back any feelings whatsoever.

At that same time I thought to myself, "Be in control and do not let any negative emotions take control over you."

"What happened to Miss Proper, always needing to hide every teardrop? Is the real me suddenly bursting out of my shell? Is my new self-emerging? Are all of these awakenings because of cancer?"

I was awakened!

8
Catch the Love Bug

The morning after the second cycle of chemo, I rolled out of bed and went to the bathroom. I felt weak and exhausted. My lack of energy went on for that entire week and it was not long before I realized I was developing a sore throat and a pain in my mouth. Every day I convinced myself the pain in my mouth would disappear by the next day, but it didn't. A low-grade fever kicked in, and I fell into total sickness. Tom was panicked. I questioned if the less aggressive chemo they promised me was doing the trick. With one incident brought on by another, one can imagine the disappointment I felt. If my doctor didn't tell me the new chemo meds would be kinder to my body, then I could have probably coped with the pain and fever. But I was angry and frustrated and disappointed, and my fever stuck to my forehead like heat on metal. Honestly scared, I wondered why all of a sudden my body was betraying me.

I did everything to make myself better. I even prohibited visitors with sick children from visiting to prevent any possible germ transportation. "So, why am I so sick?"

Tom called my nurse who then talked to my staff doctor. When the staff doctor called us at the house, I also complained of a dull pain in my kidneys.

She began questioning, "Have you been around any sick people?" Ruled out. "Do you have a burning sensation or any difficulty urinating?" Ruled out. "Is there any blood in your urine?" My urinary tract was fine.

All of my answers were an emphatic, "No!"

"You may have developed stomatitis." The doctor concluded.

"What?"

"Stomatitis is a fairly common side effect of chemotherapy," she said. "It is a condition where soreness and pain occurs in the mouth and throat. It could be accompanied by dryness and irritation, sometimes associated with an infection of some sort. The bacteria that normally live without any harm in the mouth could be causing you to have an infection. Due to a decrease in your immune function from chemotherapy, these bacteria can proliferate leading to an overgrowth in your mouth."

This was difficult for me to deal with. I was prescribed a seven-day antibiotic, and told to keep my mouth clean using the following methodology:

Mix one-fourth teaspoon of baking soda with one teaspoon of salt in one cup of warm water and rinse after each drink or meal; use a non-commercial organic tooth-paste on a soft tooth brush.

I avoided commercial rinsing agents due to their alcohol content. I was unable to chew on hard or hot foods, so I increased my juicing and drinking. I made smoothies and juices and added protein powder to guarantee I had adequate amounts of nutrients essential for healing. My fever heated my body for five long days. Though very weak, I continued eating and drinking as much as I could stomach to strengthen my ability to heal. The fever increased my determination to be even more forceful with my fight against cancer.

"This son-of-a-gun thinks by infecting my mouth and giving me a fever it can scare me? Hell no! I am here to kick cancer's ass!" And that was my promise.

When I felt feverish, I took showers to keep my body core temperature cool, sometimes twice a day. I avoided taking Tylenol; save the time my temperature exceeded one hundred point two degrees Fahrenheit. Introducing additional medications or foreign substances into my already taxed body was not on my list of priorities. During the nights, I was profusely sweating and I made certain to continue forced hydration by drinking water and nutritious juices like watermelon juice.

Additionally, I used hydrogen peroxide diluted with fifty percent water and squirted it with a syringe onto the sore spots of my mouth. I rinsed my mouth with the recommended baking soda, salt and warm water method during the day, and gargled each night before bed.

Finally after six days of a fever and a sore mouth, I managed to defeat the stomatitis and kidney pain both at once. With lots of effort, I did it; yes, I won again! Victory for Vida! I managed to save my mouth.

Shawn called, and I told him of my little victory. He frequently checked in with me, and each time I heard concern and sadness in his voice. I wished I could change everything, and told him about how I was managing to control my thoughts and rise to meet challenges with courage.

I learned the elimination of fear was a great tool contributing to my physical and emotional liveliness. I mounted an attack with a positive mind to create an offense against all obstacles.

As a female, I realized how strong women can be, as well as how patient. A compelling willpower combined with delicate emotions, sensitivity, and love is God's recipe for a woman: for a mother, grandmother, wife, sister, daughter, aunt, niece and any other female. Perhaps that is why women are the foundation of society; because it is our mission from God to be strong, to give birth, and to keep a family united. Women are the chosen ones and are uniquely phenomenal indeed.

"Is my intuitive sharpness because of cancer?"

Conscious of an increased spiritual energy, I no longer felt like damaged goods. I opened up to the universe. God created me and placed me in this world for a purpose. There is no reason I should judge myself by physical illness or any other form of material imperfection. I learned to appreciate myself even when I was bald, even when I was unable to eat, and even when I experienced any other physical dysfunction.

Personally, I was undertaking an enormous remodeling of character and finding a higher self, exploring my inner being far deeper than superficial physical changes. Superficiality was not a concern.

"No more criticizing people for being overweight and no more judging people about their fashion choices," I told myself. In essence, I no longer wanted to be such a snob.

I felt the parts of my inner depths aligning. Every day I was excited to be witness to my own growth. With each small triumph in my recovery, my soul discovered entirely new levels of being. As promises to myself, I stopped complaining about a few extra pounds here or there, stopped worrying about a few wrinkle lines on my forehead, and stopped making a fuss about a bad hair day.

Further, I promised myself to omit 'what-if' from my vocabulary and instead enjoy what I already had in my life. I planned to love more, expect less; give more without looking for the return; forgive and be more kind towards others; call my friends more often; help strangers in need.

"Is this awareness because of cancer?"

I began plotting the creation of beautiful artistic paintings. When I was only ten years old, I started oil painting. Brushing colors over canvas is still an act of passion for me. I may be considered a late bloomer, because I went back to college for the third time after sixteen years and earned another degree – one of a handful of prideful moments. As I awakened to what living really meant, I wanted to carry forward with all of my hobbies, interests and dreams. Meeting head-on with the lowest point in my life, I would not concede to letting myself or anyone else down. I played my way through a game with cancer by catching the love and prayers constantly being thrown to me from my family and friends.

Heather called me almost daily. She and I both wished she could be closer to me. She told me, "I am with you in spirit every day dear Vida."

Except when Heather called, Tom answered most of my telephone calls, because there were too many for me to handle. My heart and soul were filled by their genuine concern. I just did not have the energy to talk for very long.

I believed in the power of prayer – perseverance is all about positive energy. When every friend and family member was praying and asking others to pray, their massive energies converged into a powerful force. The whole time, I knew deep down in the depths of my heart everything was going to be all right in the end.

In retrospect, I still wonder how my husband coped with all his worries and pain. I can only imagine how difficult it must have been to be a bystander to a loved-one going through glaring pain and remain loyally supportive. No matter how hard my husband tried, he had no way of masking his worries from me. I know him too well not to see sorrow in his heart. He appreciated my dry sense of humor and laughed at the silly ways I occasionally acted. There were certainly times I acted pretty goofy during the scary days of my treatment and recovery just to cope. Perhaps my jovial personality came to him as a relief. During my treatment, I fought very hard to eliminate negative thought if it crept into my imagination.

In my philosophical mind, I thought, "If I become worried a negative vibration will resonate as a response from the universe; but if I smile, the universe will smile back to me." In the laws of universal science, same energies attract. In other words, positive attracts positive, and vice versa.

One day I was sitting at our little porch, a most relaxing and enjoyable place to be, listening to the waterfall and looking at the cherub tree. My love for gardening converted the porch to a soothing oasis. At the top of the water fountain, ivy wrapped around the structure as if holding it up and the blue and pink hydrangeas in their clay pots harmonized the atmosphere. As I sat, I carefully detected every tiny detail on all the flowers and plants. The pastel geraniums mingled over one another, climbing; the white, cupped day lilies stood erect; miniature pink roses competed for sunlight; the basil emitted a wonderful earthy fragrance. All together, nature's symphony orchestrated my amiable mood. Its song continued to play as I let go completely and tuned my soul to the pleasures of life.

Cancer really didn't matter to me. Nobody in this world has a guarantee of how long they are going to live anyway, so why worry? Instead, why not enjoy the precious moments I have to live? As I was sipping my tea and sitting in harmony, I brought my poetic notes to paper:

Love is the only contagious disease that does not need a cure!

I wish that one day it becomes epidemic and infects everybody.

I wish its cure remains unfound, and love continues spreading.

My husband, Tom spreads love throughout our home,

And it has been twenty-two long years we've been diagnosed with the love bug.

If you are not afraid of it, you may pay us a visit at home

Or online, at your own risk!

Call me selfish, but I really don't care if you catch the love bug, too.

As an artist working with colored paints, the beauty of nature's accents fascinates me. I truly believe we are all flowers in God's garden with different shapes and colors. Only He knows how to arrange his flowers in the garden of life. How boring would it be to see only one kind of flower in the garden, only one standard color or shape? Conceivably that is why God created everyone differently, to excite us with the splendor of variety.

Tom uses the organic basil, rosemary, mint and tarragon we have growing for his cooking. We end up saving a bit of money, as he prefers to incorporate our homegrown fresh herbs, garlic and lemon in most of his dishes, eliminating the need for extra salt or fat flavorings. I am indisputably blessed to be sharing life with him. My goodness, he made an immeasurable difference with the preparation of exciting meals to encourage my demoralized appetite and increased my well being during the phases of my recovery.

Tom is famous for his creative cooking and our friends believe he is truly a gifted chef. His cooking possesses healing qualities and could serve to help more people than just myself. Though his cooking has remained within the confines of our home kitchen, the flavor is so good his meals could endow an entire restaurant. His dishes could uphold a reputation of being the most prestigious gourmet health cuisine; I do not know of any restaurant to dish up nutritious creations like Tom's.

Sometimes he teased me about how easily I responded to him when a conversation turned over about food. He said I did not take as much interest in any other subjects and thought they were inferior to and not as exciting as food. I could not take fault for having a man that frequently talked about food and for taking a keen interest in what he was saying about it. But he will definitely have to take fault if I gained weight from eating his meals, though.

9
Organic Happy Meal

I had a slight weight gain during my treatment. Thus far, however, my doctors told me whatever I was doing in regards to diet was working well. They had no idea Tom dedicated more hours in the kitchen to my nutrition than any one else on my entire medical team did to my treatment. Natural organic foods and a positive perspective deserve credit for my healing progressions.

Just a nibble of common sense may be required to wonder if health problems arise from foods people are eating. Chew on this: about twenty or more years ago, there was a popular illustrated television commercial with a catchy song, "We are what we eat, from our head down to our feet." It's true, we are what we eat; so do you want to be a sausage, or as cool as a cucumber?

I have always been health conscious, and an advocate of eating healthy. I have seen chemotherapy patients eating French fries and other fast foods for their lunch, washing down a 'what-ever burger' with a can of soda.

"Do people lack awareness of what they are doing to themselves?" A friend told me of how lung cancer patients at Sloan Kettering cancer center in New York stand on the sidewalk with their IV pole, smoking cigarettes. I was appalled and speechless.

In the same light, I was seriously frightened when I saw cancer patients eating fast food and sipping soda. Proper nutritional advice should be a highlighted branch of patient health education.

Now honestly people: Is it really a good idea to have a fast-food restaurant in a hospital? How can doctors advise patients about nutrition in the same building where fast food is sold? The concept does not make sense. I just do not understand how a fast-food restaurant can be established in the same hospital as patients suffering with diabetes, cardiovascular disease, or cancer. Isn't that insult to injury?

I watched as patients wearing hospital gowns purchased burgers and fries and soda in the hospital where I was being treated. I summoned every bit of restraint in my body to hold back from gently tapping on their shoulder to conduct a brief educational tutorial about ways to change their diet from fast food to truly nutritious food. I wish people recognized that eating a boiled egg and a banana versus fried greasy foods and soda costs nearly the same at the grocery store. To their dismay they shall realize that the affects of grease and sugar affect every organ in the body and are extremely high taxes the body cannot afford.

In part, I believe I survived cancer because Tom filled me with organic and delicious foods, including juicing. He also fed and nurtured my soul with his love.

As a doctor, I always advised my patients about the importance of a well balanced diet. Tom and I have taken a special liking for juicing and nutrition because we realized how much it lends a hand in healing processes.

I remember when I was a student we performed a laboratory experiment growing bacteria in a sugar agar dish, then compared it with bacterial growth in a non-sugar lab dish. After three days my classmates and I checked the two different dishes to find the bacteria *thriving* in the sugary environment.

When I was first diagnosed with cancer, macrobiotic cooking was the style Tom adopted for all of my meals. In macrobiotic cooking everything is cooked with low heat, no animal fat is recommended. Great sources of information about macrobiotic cooking are available online of course, for those who take an interest. Sea vegetables (sold dry in *Whole Foods*® *Market*) whole grain cereals, brown rice, and a variety of legumes (beans) are used in moderation. Nutrition is based on balance, specifically in regards to acid and alkaline food intakes. For example, vegetables such as eggplant, tomatoes, mushrooms and the like are considered nightshade-grown and are discouraged during cancer treatment. Sugars along with refined and processed foods were prohibited.

My husband used mostly fish, fresh fruits and vegetables in his cooking. Nuts made great snacks. I found it amazing how the right foods enhanced my energy levels and boosted my ability to recovery from my treatments.

During chemotherapy I was unable to continue eating one hundred percent macrobiotic cooking because my appetite was crushed by chemo. I had to eat anything appealing to my depleted appetite. I lived on iced-cold beverages and organic homemade banana pudding. However, I did continue to consume foods prepared through slow or low-heat cooking methods. The low fat and sugar-free foods remained the same in my diet.

Due to the significant decrease in my desire to eat, I was very fussy at times and had a hard time consuming foods, most noticeably the first two days following chemo treatments. A high protein shake was a good choice for me to keep my body strong. The shake was made using either rice milk or low fat milk or almond milk combined with frozen fruits like peaches, strawberries and fresh bananas, as well as one scoop of protein powder. Crushed ice made the shakes easier to swallow. One scoop of protein powder supplied ten grams of protein and if I wanted a greater amount, then another scoop was added.

Some mornings my husband made egg white omelets with pesto sauce and toasted wheat pita bread. Yum, the omelets were absolutely delicious!

The key to tolerating food was a smaller portion of food in a higher frequency, rather than a large amount all at once. To set a baseline, I learned to listen to my body's needs to determine what I really liked eating. Boy, my appetite was so particular, it was worse than when I was pregnant with my son. I disliked foods I previously enjoyed, and initially it was awfully difficult to find something to eat. On the worst days, even if food had been delivered from heaven it would have tasted like cardboard. I had a strange taste in my mouth that made eating a chore and all I wanted to eat was something extremely cold to sooth my sore mouth. Tom always made something tasty so I was never starving.

The days when I had a better appetite were the days just prior to the next chemo treatment. Usually, I had high protein and colorful meals to optimize my energy and stay strong through the next treatment. I drank water, water, water like a fish-fish-fish! During the days of chemotherapy and two days following, I drank about a gallon of water each day to flush my kidneys clean of medicine. On an average day, I drank about ten to twelve glasses of juice, water or other liquids. Because they are normally loaded with sugars, I did not drink pre-packed or can juice, no thank you. It was scary reading the labels of factory-made drinks and seeing the high sugar contents. The one pre-packed drink I did consume was oxygenated or spring water, as well as the variety of milks in the shakes.

Out of curiosity, one day in a health food market I decided to check the ingredients of a popular brand of energy and protein bars and discovered an extensive list of sugars on the labels: corn syrups, diglycerides, triglycerides, and canes.

"Health bar? Sugar does not equate to health." I thought.

After I was diagnosed, I began the habit of reading every single label. Though time consuming, I became used to knowing the items or brands reliable for *real* nutrition. After a few weeks, shopping did not take quite as long.

10
Two Green Apples Fell From the Tree

As my chemotherapy was close to being finished, I became lethargic and impatient. I felt so sluggish I thought there was no life left in my body. Nothing was interesting to me. I had to guide and push my body with the power of my mind to make it through every day. To empower myself from within, I turned my attention to my higher self through meditation and visualizations of my dreams.

I said to myself, "I wish to have peace of mind and perfect health." I visualized the conception of a cancer center with every thing that would help people to heal. So real in its form, the vivid image truly distracted my mind from worry. My main challenge to fill the void cancer created in my life was replacing physical weakness and pain with wonderful thoughts, feelings and experiences.

Post-chemotherapy, my body was motionless or asleep for several days, my spirit elsewhere. The best I could do was read a book or watch television. Sometimes I would wake up in the middle of the night and walk around the house like a zombie. Other patients I knew undergoing the same treatment did not have this experience. Some complained of nausea and vomiting while others were able to go to work the very next day after chemotherapy. Just as I've said, people are different.

My husband always asked me to wake him if I could not sleep so we could watch television together. He simply wanted to keep me company. Since I could not trust my mood at any given moment, I never woke him. I tried eating fruit or having a drink, and then played on the computer or as I mentioned, flipped through late night television programs. Mostly I kept quiet and tried to visualize all the good things; sometimes I wrote in my journal.

In my writing, I prayed for patients with more severe cases than mine, asking God to help them regain the strength to recover. In addition to extending healing energy to others, writing prayers helped me to feel more focused on my own recovery as well. Anytime when there was a difficulty in my life, I thought about people with more severe circumstances than my own as a reminder that Tom and I were not the only ones in the world with problems.

Soon the third cycle of my chemotherapy approached. I was praying to God I would not suffer as badly as the last chemotherapy cycle. Sitting in the waiting area, I knew, as always, it took time before I would hear my name called. I was accustomed to waiting. I patiently read my book to kill the time, but I could not ignore the people sitting around me. As I looked over the top of my book around the crowded room, scanning the faces, I spotted a thin young woman. She spoke to me with her broken English.

"I am waiting for my chemo session. I feel fine but my doctor told me the cancer spread to my lung and liver now." She was ignorant of the denotation of what she was saying, unaware that metastatic cancer meant she was regressing. But I was wholeheartedly disturbed to hear her cancer was metastasizing. I tried to offer her information about nutrition. What else could I possibly do for her?

Patients were forced to wait many long painful hours in the hospital before being treated. Frustration, grief, sorrow, and poverty plastered across all of their faces.

After every visit to the Oncology department, I went back home with more emotional pain at what I witnessed than physical pain for my own illness. Had I never visited the county hospital, I would have never known that level of disparity existed in peoples' lives.

Normally I waited more than one hour before I was called for the routine of blood work and physical exam. I would give a blood sample and while waiting for the lab results, a nurse checked my weight, my vital signs and so forth. That day my waiting time exceeded four hours. I was exhausted and wondered what was taking so long.

Tom tried to comfort me, "Be patient, Sweetheart. Let's wait just a little longer. I am sure there is a reason for the delay."

I finally ran out of patience and went to the front desk.

The receptionist simply said, "Your scheduled appointment has been changed."

The wrath of my anger said, "I signed-in when I first entered four hours ago. Why wasn't I told about a change of my schedule then?" This was unacceptable to me "Can I speak with the floor supervisor?" I asked.

When the supervisor arrived I was in tears. I felt ignored and mistreated. I didn't know what they were thinking, failing to communicate a change in plans. Was there no regard to the emotional well being of a cancer patient, forced to be kept waiting uninformed of a change in plans, disrespected and battered by indolence?

"Don't I have enough to handle? How dare they?"

The supervisor apologized and mentioned that my assigned doctor had a change in schedule.

She said, "Somehow she forgot to report her change to the front desk."

The oncology clinic had only one day per week for breast oncology patients to visit their assigned doctors.

The supervisor informed me, "Since our clinic is affiliated with the medical university we are short of doctors today. We are dependant on the university's schedule."

She shook her head, "I am so sorry. I started working here about a month ago, and I am trying to make things more organized." She said they had more patients to treat than they could handle.

I did not have any other choice other than to return the following week when they could schedule me again.

The following week after I receive my last chemotherapy, I returned home and I was doing fine the first day. After a restful night, I felt the medicine begin kicking in. A friend from out of town was staying at our house to offer Tom a break from the kitchen and assist with taking care of me. Even though I was feeling low on energy, my friend and I were still able to enjoy each other's company. From the living room, I overheard her on the telephone saying how well I seemed to be doing. She must have spoke too soon, because the next day I fell into an acute episode of weakness and it took me about five days to recover. Comparatively, this treatment made me brutally feeble, but I was still not vomiting and was still grateful.

Every day I woke up with the unyielding hope of having a better day than the one before. My energy level went up, down, down further, up again, down, up and I really could not predict its patterns. All I knew, I was thankful my mouth wasn't sore and I didn't have a fever anymore.

My strength abounded with the thought that chemo was finally over. I regarded chemotherapy as a necessary process of debugging from cancer. As an analogy to my beautiful rose bushes in the garden, if they were not heavily sprayed with de-bugging chemical agents, they died from the attack of insects. The chemical treatment allowed the chance for them to bloom again, just as chemotherapy provided me a chance to blossom. Okay, my attitude was changing for the better. Bitterness was not supposed to be part of treatment; it was not good for anyone, and not good for me. So I stayed positive.

Six weeks after chemo treatment ended, radiation therapy was set to begin, and I went to meet with my appointed radiation oncologist. She walked into the treatment room where I sat waiting for her. Very friendly, her sweetness comforted me. I told her I knew everything about her.

"I Googled you!" I said to her, and she smiled.

She said modestly, "Oh, I am glad you did." I discovered she had over eighteen years of experience in her field of practice, and had a stint as an assistant professor.

Examining my right breast, she said with slight apprehension, "I am concerned with this lump in your right breast. Let's perform another mammogram before moving forward with your radiation therapy."

I was shocked since my most recent mammogram four months prior had not revealed any suspicious findings. Astonished by the set back, I wondered in fear if I would have to go through chemo again.

"Will I be able to survive another round of chemo? Well, I have to do what I have to do," I thought.

Welcome to the reality show of the fight against cancer.

The mammogram was performed and the result was luckily negative. I was back to proceeding with radiation therapy. The preparation started by mapping the affected left breast. The doctor took measurements and x-rayed my breast. At the same time, the radiology technician made a permanent marking on my skin referred to as tattooing. The tattoo is actually a conglomerate of small dots of ink at the focal point where the radiation beam should aim during each session. Having the tattoo makes it easier for the performing technician to know the exact location to treat.

My treatment plan for radiation was set to be six and half weeks every day, except weekends. Each session lasted about ten minutes and it seemed like a breeze compared to chemotherapy.

After four weeks of radiation, I started feeling a burning sensation on my nipple. The skin near the nipple discolored like a sunburn. I applied pure Aloe-Vera gel at the burn site after each treatment, and carried a small container of the gel in my handbag to use when I changed from hospital gown to my clothes. I also applied it a few other times throughout the day to cool the burning sensation on my skin. At the end of my radiation therapy my nipple was so sore I tried to keep it from rubbing against my clothing.

My eagerness to make it through radiation therapy, the last of my treatments, and to carry on with life occupied my mind. I filled empty nights of sleeplessness by planning my future and creating lectures about breast cancer awareness to present to various colleges and schools. The public needs to learn about my firsthand experience as a terminally ill patient without insurance. As a patient with an extensive education in the medical fields of nursing and chiropractic, I felt I had a unique perspective of the treatment offered in a county hospital verses any other type of medical center.

On one level, I believed my treatments might have been slightly easier for me if I was not subjected to witnessing how people around me suffered through their illness in poverty. My soul was disturbed at how they could not even afford a meal to nourish themselves. On another level, perhaps the realization that their life threatening situations were not much different from mine served as motivation for me to survive, so at some point I might be poised to offer help in some way. I felt a sense of obligation to find ways to assist other patients in need.

There were already many foundations for research in this country making remarkable discoveries to create better treatment protocols. Women needed help in a variety of other ways. But there was more to the needs of a patient than better techniques of chemotherapy and radiation. As an eyewitness I tell you, women brought their children to chemotherapy with them because they could not afford a baby sitter. Their dresses tattered and torn, I saw expressions of lost hope on their faces.

The idea of establishing a foundation to financially assist breast cancer patients took over my thoughts. Having seen despair in the lives of others, I wanted to extend a good will offering to women dealing with this devastating disease. My breast cancer foundation could assist disadvantaged or uninsured women with a lack of sufficient funds. The foundation could be set up to assist with paying for treatments or in the very least provide financial support for every day living expenses. I envisioned a cancer center to facilitate another level of healing during and after a patient's treatments. I envisioned a place people could eat organic and healthy foods, enjoy listening to music, meditate, and be engaged in activities to fill their body and soul.

I planned and planned and planned, one idea after another. Productively and positively utilized my precious time during the long nights to conceptualize how to generate funds for this foundation.

I had an idea, and once again, it involved food.

During the dark hours of the night when I could not sleep, especially during the late summer months, I started thinking about biscotti endlessly, cooking up a completely organic recipe to sell and raise funds for my newly-imagined breast cancer foundation. Six years ago, I started sending my homemade biscotti to friends as part of a Christmas basket gift.

"Could my biscotti help manifest my dream?"

I loved biscotti; this Italian cookie has been my all-time favorite. For as long as I can remember, I enjoyed it with tea, coffee, milk and even on its own. My obsession for this cookie combined with the passion and love I put into baking it made for a wonderful treat for others to enjoy.

On the days I felt physically strong I baked, and then sent samples of my biscotti, not just to family and friends but also to professional organizations. Tom helped by delivering samples of my cranberry-walnut and almond-orange biscotti to *Whole Foods*® *Market* and other bakeries for tasting. With a steadfast determination, I sought feed-back for my developments.

I hoped through the combined sales of my biscotti and my book, enough funds would be generated to meet the needs of as many women as possible.

Rather than focusing on just myself, I began planning more lofty ideas on how to help others. The efforts I put into my work, gave me profound pleasure money could never afford.

"I have great ideas and I know what needs to be done; but where do I begin," I asked myself.

Two beautiful green apples stuck as an image in my head for days and nights on end. I did not fully grasp the lasting mental impression for quite a while.

One night I analyzed why the image continually flashed through my mind. In many cultures apples are a symbol for health, and green a color of peace and healing. I assumed the digit two was the representation of female breasts. I said to myself, "Maybe this is the answer to my question. Is this a potential name for my cancer foundation?"

And *2 Green Apples* came into fruition, the logo wishing every woman on the face of the planet to have two healthy breasts.

My healing philosophy is strongly rooted in the belief that positive thoughts and feelings have a positive influence on the body. Say, for example, a patient had the most proficient doctors working with them, and utilized the most advanced technologies in medicine for their treatment plan, neither of those factors would allow for the patient to respond favorably, unless the patient actually empowered their own healing with convicted belief in their ability to survive. I speak from personal experience. Hope was my most powerful instrument in the process of healing.

As soon as I awoke during those nights and before I even left my bed, unorganized thoughts inundated my head on the pillow.

"What am I going to do? What if things do not work out? How can I start a non-profit foundation? Where can I sell my cookies? What should I do today?" Sidetracked confusion and worry tormented me. You may be familiar with this insomniatic mind pattern of waking and worrying, where the right side of the brain wanders off in thought.

I figured if I closely monitored my own thought patterns, I would be able to move forward and focus on being productive.

"If I am meant to die at this point in my life, panic is certainly not going to elongate my life." I analyzed my situation. "Why not leave a lasting footprint and memory of myself on earth by doing something remarkable?"

I became so involved with writing and baking biscotti for my *2 Green Apples* foundation; the last thing on my mind was worrying about breast cancer recovery. The power of positive thinking made an amazing different in helping to quiet the noise of fearful thoughts polluting my brain.

I forcefully shifted my thoughts to stop thinking only about myself, regardless of whether or not the thoughts about *me* were good or otherwise. My full recovery from breast cancer was becoming a more likely reality; I wanted to create my version of a cancer foundation for the life-affirming goal of helping others.

I talked with everyone I knew about my plan to start a breast cancer network. My friend Heather was not excessively fond of my nonstop efforts. She was more concerned about my wellness and thought I needed to save my energy for healing and my own wellness. However, I felt like a Mack truck speeding down a hill unstoppable. I had a mission.

I began planning the first fundraising event for by creating a silent auction. Tom sent written invitations and group E-vites through mass e-mailings spreading a notice of our tremendous intentions with the auction. Using his graphic designing skills, Tom ingeniously designed a professional quality label and logo for the biscotti. Furthermore, he worked with food laboratories to gain an FDA approval for the nutritional factors of our recipe.

Local businesses made monetary donations to help pay for the dinner served. Some guests donated items to be auctioned. I personally donated a large portion of my jewelry collection, many of our antiques and other collectibles, and a few oil paintings from my portfolio. Further, we turned our home into a small biscotti factory with family and friends helping to prepare for the event. Together we baked hundreds of boxes and bags of organic low-fat biscotti, professionally wrapped and labeled with the foundation's new name and logo: *2 Green Apples, inc.*

Sitting in front of my vanity mirror preparing to hold my first fundraising dinner for the foundation, I was pumped with excitement the roof of my house had trouble containing. It had been a while since my last session of radiation therapy and Tom thought I needed to slow down a bit. At eight o'clock, people would begin to show up – about one hundred and twenty guests were expected.

"Things are happening just like I planned during the sleepless nights of my treatment," I thought.

I was still wearing a wig. I used eyeliner and eye shadow so my eyes wouldn't look like fish eyes; I had no eyelashes on my eyelids. My brows were only about fifty percent flourishing, "but not a problem – I am good with make-up." As a matter of fact, my painting skills came in very handy to illuminate my face, accentuating its features. I pulled on my pink outfit, and tried to find a lipstick to match its soft color. As they say: "Look good, feel good!" Make-up helped not only to make me feel better about myself, but also helped people around me to feel more comfortable. If they were thinking, "She does not look sick at all; she looks GREAT!" then that was the energy I received from them, greatness.

A few minutes before the eight o'clock hour, the door-bell rang, and our guests began arriving. The weather was pleasant so Tom opened the double-doors from our living room to our patio to diffuse the people packing into our home. To my surprise we had a remarkable response from our community and the event turned out rather tastefully. The biscotti generated the most sales for the night. Minus deductions for expenses, the funds earned from the auction proceeded directly to my breast cancer foundation.

During the auction, I set up accounts at three different venues to sell my biscotti: a local bank, a private medical center, and a country club.

"The biscotti business will only survive with multiple vendors selling them," I thought.

I began visiting coffee shops and health food stores with more samples of biscotti, and hoped to provide exposure for *2 Green Apples, inc.* Over the next few months, a few hundred dollars worth of biscotti was sold. It was not easy for me to continually bake and sell biscotti at the same time going under cancer treatment. No matter how great the product, promoting it required a large marketing platform. My goals were greater than what I could handle on my own. Our oven was only large enough to bake enough cookies to fulfill small orders. In addition, our monthly electric bill was rising. Although I was working very hard, the expenses exceeded the income.

By Christmas 2007, I raised four thousand dollars. I thought I should start small and give the money to women at the county hospital for the holiday season.

I went to the main office for the American Cancer Society at the county hospital and asked for contact information of breast cancer patients. However, my request could not be granted. Because of patient confidentiality, they would not release names or addresses.

"Hmm," I thought, as I turned to leave, "How can I distribute these donations to patients? I don't feel quite right about handing envelops of cash to people in the waiting room of the breast oncology ward."

As I left the office, a couple of bald women like myself approached me and began following me down the hall. They said they overheard my conversation and thought they could help me allocate the funds. With the help of those two women (I don't even remember their names), I had more than twenty names and addresses of breast cancer patients to send anonymous donations. I put cash in envelopes, and on my way to the post office, I divided the cash evenly between twenty-four stamped envelopes and dropped them in the mail. When I returned from the post office, I realized I actually gave myself the most wonderful Christmas present ever by giving to others.

11
County Hospital

J ust when I was almost done with what I thought to be the biggest challenge of my life – that is to say, fighting for survival – something even more devastating competed and turned out to be the most challenging period of all of my struggles.

As the backdrop leading up to this point, over the course of the start up period for Tom's corporation overseas, he worked almost an entire year without drawing an income. He poured money into the hope of a return on his investment. As a consequence of seeking to lift his business ideas off the ground, he drew from our savings accounts to pay for business and living expenses without earning a dime. The endeavor seemed very promising and he kept working on his brand new company, in a brand new country with the expectation of earning a profitable fortune.

Before we knew it, a year passed since our move. Tom continued planting seeds to set the groundwork for his business, struggling for foundation. Poor Tom did all he could think of, but was acting like a desperate gambler in an expensive casino spending his last dollars for the chance to hit the jackpot with his business. Discouraged, he reached the bottom point of staying home and staring at the television, pretending everything was fine. He wanted to protect me from knowing his despair. However, I was entirely aware of the depths of his troubles. I could feel it.

Tom has always been a workaholic. By saying that, I respectfully mean he worked twenty-four hours every day of his life, and our stint overseas was the first time in our marriage I had to work full-time to subsidize our family. The income from my chiropractic practice paid for all of our living expenses. I was enjoying my practice and loved my patients, but when I saw the disappointment Tom experienced from his miscalculated business decisions, I was very disturbed. We had intended to save a chunk of money for our retirement; but instead our path was leading us in the opposite direction towards poverty.

As a reminder, let me point out that was during the time I was encountering my own personal changes with menopause. Masses of problems from every direction came after the two of us. I had never imagined life's setbacks would smother us as if being engulfed in quick sand. Neither of us ever faced systemic impoverishment – as I called it.

Our entire lives were lived virtually in the lap of luxury, so to speak, traveling around the world and spending as we wished. I guess the time had come for us to experience another side of the coin.

In a search to regain his financial losses, as I mentioned, Tom ended up leaving without seeing that fortune to pickup with the business offer in Connecticut.

When Tom and I moved back to the Dallas, it took us several months to become settled. There were many arrangements to make, including the relocation to Texas, finding a new home, and reconstructing our lives.

In the first few months of being in Dallas, I was so busy there was not a second for me to think of anything other than settling in. Tom was occupied with creating yet another business venture, and neither of us were paying enough attention to our spending. The remainder of our savings trickled out over so many things, and became depleted by the expenses of living.

When I was first diagnosed with cancer, we were unable to acquire health insurance for two major reasons. Firstly, the very obvious reason was my terminal illness. Yes, because I had cancer. Insurance companies do not insure people with major pre-existing sickness like cancer.

Secondly, we were both unemployed. Desperate to find a solution to save my life, we felt helpless. Never in our wildest dreams had we imagined this nightmare would happen to us, or anyone else for that matter. Really, I never even thought it was possible to drain our bank accounts completely dry, become terminally ill with a cancerous disease, and then be rejected by health insurance companies – the entire world turned against me; that's how I felt. Every moment was crucial to find a way to treat my breast cancer.

With the recommendation of a few close friends in the medical field, I applied to the county hospital known for its advanced medical technology. I was one of the fifty some-odd million people in the United States without health insurance. Finally, after filling-out dozens of pages of application forms at the county hospital, I was admitted. In regular everyday life, I never went to places I did not feel comfortable. At the county hospital I felt like I was on a separate planet from everyone else, and unable to relate with the people. Passers-by stared at me, with glaring eyes. I was used to expressing my outgoing personality, talking with people around me and meeting new people. However, I did not fit into this hospital's environment; I did not even feel welcomed and only interacted with the medical staff.

So as not to attract attention, I tended to my outward appearance. I felt liable for how I presented myself and did not want to be over dressed. I was always anxious to be done with my treatment so I could leave the hospital.

The day I set foot into a county hospital was a day I never thought I would live to see. I saw desperately poor families, people who were illiterate and most of them spoke very little or broken English. Plus, there were prisoners with handcuffs being escorted by police officers through the halls.

"Oh my Lord! Why do I deserve this anguish?" I wished for an answer. "I used to be the one taking care of patients with all my heart and soul. How did I end up a sick patient unable to afford to get better? Wake-me-up; wake-me-up. Wake me up from this bad dream! Please!!"

On the up side, perhaps being financially troubled had an unexpected silver lining when it came to premium care being accessible to me. Despite my humiliation, I was treated by some of the best specialist in the country. Also, by coming in contact with people I never before had been so close to, I was taught many, many valuable life lessons. Through my experiences at that hospital, I learned aspects of human pain and suffering I may have never learned otherwise.

When I was walking onto the elevator to go up to the breast oncology department for one of my first chemo treatments, there was a female cancer patient: bald, pale, and tired, just like me. I saw her walk into the hospital's cafeteria next to the elevator. She stopped and looked at the menu, turning the saliva over in her mouth as she licked her lips. Wearing a hospital gown, she appeared as if she did not have any money to buy lunch. As a kind gesture, I treated her hunger with a sandwich and fruit.

Each day I returned from the hospital for my treatment, I thought about all of the starving people living in our country known to the world as one of the wealthiest, the same country that sends aid to foreign nations despite the fact that fellow citizens are hungry and without food.

Over all, the worst day of all my terror was the day I was rushed to the hospital. It was ten in the morning, three days after one of my first chemo treatment when I returned home after my morning walk and felt a sharp pain in my spine. Trying to ignore my pain, I sat down on an armchair with my legs rested on the ottoman; after a minute or two the pain grew worse, like a stabbing of a knife into my back. When Tom saw a curtain of whiteness fall over my face, sweat beading across my brow, he sat down on the ottoman and watched over me. With each breath, the mortifying pain intensified and I began screaming. Not knowing what to do, Tom gave me a Hydrocodone, the painkiller prescribed by my oncologist. After five minutes the pain cut in half, but we had no idea what was causing it. I could barley move without screaming in pain.

Tom called my doctor and she insisted for me to go immediately to the hospital. Although I was an existing patient with a mammoth patient file, when I arrived to the hospital they asked me to go to the Emergency Room.

In the ER I was treated as if I was a *new* patient. An intern guided me through an entry questionnaire, a case history and then a complete physical exam – a most annoying and lengthy process for an existing patient. The entire time I was in severe pain. When she was through with the entry procedures, she asked me to wait for the next available floor doctor. The emergency room personnel had no way of accessing my patient file of six months; and the irony of the situation, when I became upset and complained about it, they plainly said, "Sorry."

Though a large and advanced hospital with high tech equipment and a wide-range of personnel, it was not very patient friendly nor personable.

"Is this a legitimate expectation, to be treated with *care*; or am I asking too much?" I pondered.

Each time when I was sent for a different consultation with a different nurse – every single time – they started from ground zero.

Finally, after four hours in the hallway on a stretcher, the doctor came by to say, "There is nothing we can do at this time because it's Saturday, and there are not any oncologist on board here today."

"Aaaahhh!!" I was shrieking on the inside. "It was my Oncologists' strong suggestion to go to the ER in the first place, because she felt my case was urgent enough for immediate care. Now they are sending me away without attending to my intense pain?" I was left dangling and dishonored, untreated.

The nurse said, "I am going to give you a painkiller that you can take until tomorrow when the MRI center is open and the oncologist is available to see you." She was going to write a prescription for more painkillers, the same ones I was already taking. Tom pulled the container of Hydro-codone from his pocket and showed the doctor. What a disgrace.

The lack of communication within the hospital's system stemmed from the ER's inability to access my patient file. Why would a doctor write a duplicate prescribe of medication I was already taking? That seemed negligent. And why should a patient have to go through so many repeated and unnecessary steps, where time could have been more productively spent on trying to ease my unbearable pain?

The cause of the shocking pain in my spine remained a mystery.

12
A Journal of Hope

It was still the beginning of my lengthy journey of reaching my lofty ambitions of having a sustaining foundation for breast cancer patients. As John F Kennedy once said in accordance with the ancient Chinese proverb, "A journey of a thousand miles must begin with a single step." I hoped other women in the future would continue the development of my new ideas with the foundation, and hoped it would live on to be a beneficial financial resource for breast cancer victims.

I kept a notebook available at my bedside for the moments when ideas came fresh into my mind and recorded them in their pristine form. I wrote notes of encouragement for myself.

"I am almost there! I am done with the tests and surgery, and most of my treatments are behind me. Hang in there, Vida! Although it may be tough, I am going to survive long enough to share my experiences of winning this fight."

The act of writing placed me in a position of strength, because I looked forward with vision. I was not sure how it began exactly, but my determined drive was very powerful. Today you are reading a book made of all those notes written through the nights – my raw expressions in the loneliest moments of my fear, the desperate moments of hope, and the turnover of my dreams as I trucked forward with living.

I wrote, "I believe everybody's life is an unread book. Each individual has a unique life experience and their own story to tell. No matter how many books about breast cancer are on the shelves, my individual experience is different and might serve to benefit a woman with breast cancer. I will write to them; I write *for* them."

Christmas was fast approaching and I was as excited as a little girl. A decorative light cheerfully illuminated neighborhood houses, wreathes, and garland. Shopping malls buzzed with the holiday spirit. I was soon going to celebrate the end of my major treatments, and this was a very special Christmas to my family and to me. My son, Shawn and his two friends planned to join us from Florida.

I busily decorated my house and shopped for presents. Everything seemed so festive, I almost forgot about cancer. A mind distracted with positive thoughts and actions again kept me so full of joy there was no space left for cancer. Because of being engulfed by the season, I stopped meditating on a regular basis, though. Deep down I was a little uncomfortable with the shift in my prioritizing, but I tried to meditate when I could fit it in. I felt a bit guilty for not spending the few crucial minutes each day to set my mind straight with meditative focus.

I promised myself as soon as the holiday season ended I would go back to my favorable routines. There was also something else I needed to do.

After Christmas and the New Year, I decided it was time to pay a visit to my family in the Middle East. Throughout the entire time I was going through treatment, I never alerted them of my situation with breast cancer. It was difficult to keep from telling them, but my decision was to tell my parents and siblings in person and at the right time. The oceans between us were too large for them to be able to come to the States; and the political state of affairs made it nearly impossible for them to acquire a visa to travel into the United States. So what purpose would I serve by revealing the bad news when they could not be next to me? All I would do by sharing the horror with my family would create anxious concern resulting in a negative energy flow of parental and sibling worry.

It had been a year since I was diagnosed with breast cancer. My friends had differing opinions about my decision to keep my illness a secret from my family most disagreed. One close friend however, was very supportive. She understood my position because she lost her mother to colon cancer and at the time her mother was living in England. I personally remember how disturbed she felt by being so far away and unable to be with her mother to offer care and support in a proper way.

Both excited and nervous to see my family, the day arrived and I was on the plane – millions of thoughts flying through my muddled mind. I was happy and full of joy, though. I could not believe I was well again. But it was for real and I could live like a regular person. I could fly anywhere in the world. I did not have to go to the hospital every day anymore; my God, my new reality.

My hair had grown about one inch long. Fairly skinny and insignificantly pale, I had an energy level like a healthy individual. The scar remains at the right upper center of my chest below my clavicle bone from the Mediport where they injected the chemotherapy medication. I didn't want to wear a top with an opening around my chest to draw attention to the scar. Since it was winter, I wore a sweater and the immediate exposure of my scar on the day of my arrival was not a concern.

Thirty hours of travel between driving to the airport and flying, I finally made it to my homeland very exhausted.

I thought, "Maybe it was a little too early for me to take such a long trip?" But I was without a doubt desperate to make this trip, and excited to see my family. The heavy load I carried with the secret of my cancer needed to be lifted from my shoulders.

At the end of the terminal, my brother was waiting for me with a beautiful bouquet of flowers. He was alone. I insisted the entire family did not come to the airport so I would have enough room in the car for my luggage – mainly filled with gifts for everyone. We had not seen each other for over two years.

My brother is not usually very talkative, but during the car-ride home we talked back and forth non-stop. We missed each other so badly. Just over a year younger than me, my brother works in the construction business, mostly building new homes. He is my only brother and because of his reliability, he was assigned as the power of attorney on my behalf, if ever needed. I trust him with all of my heart. He described all of the details about his current project, a new house he was building in town, and spoke of the group of people he was working with.

Before we knew it, we arrived at our parent's house. I spent an entire week with them before I was even close to ready to reveal my secret. The happiness to unite as a family was too precious to be ruined by my disturbing news.

One afternoon, as I was lying down on my large king sized bed reading, Nasrin, one of my sisters, walked in my room and threw her self atop of the bed.

"Stop reading, Vida; spend some time with us. Isn't that why you are home?" Nasrin asked. In her late thirties, Nasrin is my youngest sister. She is a law school graduate and can speak English fluently.

"This book is so spiritual and inspiring!" I said, folding it closed over my finger to mark the page. As we began talking about the contents of the book, our two other sisters, Nahid and Nooshin, joined our bed party. Ever since we were children, my sisters and I had a custom of lying on the bed together to gossip and laugh. It was an endearing way for us to reconnect. Very close in age, the four of us have always remained intimately and immeasurably connected with one another.

Nahid, is a retired nurse in her late forties, and the closest in age to me. Her husband was a pilot trained by the United States Navy. Because she lost her husband during the war against Iraq, Nahid was forced to raise her children alone. Her funny personality and personal integrity provided her with the strength to carry on after the loss of her late husband. Everybody loves her to death and thinks of her as the queen of gossip.

Our middle sister, Nooshin is a librarian: brilliant and beautiful inside and out. She recommends many great books, and acts as the family's advisor and distributor of quality literature. Our family is a group of book-lovers, thanks to my mother initially, but now everyone always asks Nooshin's opinion about a book before reading it. Nooshin is currently learning English from her young son and doing quite well with her progressions with studying the language.

As the four of us were lying on the bed, Nahid twirling Nasrin's hair with her finger and Nooshin's head resting on the pillow next to mine, I started translating a chapter of the book I was reading. In my translation, I interjected an explanation of the power of the mind and positive thinking, and so forth. As I continued reading, all three sisters became intrigued and were so inquisitive about the book for the rest of the day. They hovered over me and followed me to be sure they were with me when I started reading again. At any rate, my interpretation of the book was a great exercise to prepare and lead up to the news I was about to report.

Finally, I felt ready to reveal my secret. We called our brother into the room and I told all four of my siblings at once. As I was telling my gruesome story of prevailing victory, they each lovingly touched me. I described everything about my past year from start to finish: diagnosis, treatment and recovery, with an emphasis of how my positive attitude and determination to heal helped me win my fight against cancer. All of us entangled in a group huddle, it was an emotional scene of tears, hugs and support.

Their support and encouragement meant the world to me, and I felt relieved to finally tell them. They were all so happy to know I was healthy again and admitted they would have felt miserable if they found out while I was so far away. Thankful for the opportunity to hear my story in person, they confirmed that they would have been extremely troubled by not being able to be with me during my cancer treatment.

Do you see what I mean about creating a negative energy flow?

Still keeping the pact to this day, my siblings and I consented not to share my story with our parents. My mother and father simply could not handle it. Devastating news about their first child having cancer is not needed to aggravate their old age and poor health. In their minds, a cancer diagnosis was nothing short of a death sentence. People from the Middle East are easily hurt when it comes to the bond amongst family members, and one of them suffering. With an epic sensitivity and an immense love for one another, their emotions may have spiraled out of control. I did not want to be a cause of pain, not in the least.

Visiting time with the family came to a close, and it was time to return to Dallas where Tom waited for me. My son and my friends back in the States were not pleased I took the trip because of the war in the Middle East, but thank goodness everything went smoothly and I returned safely.

13
Postal Delivery

The jet lag had me bumping along slowly gaining pace to the routines of my daily life with Tom. It was very refreshing to have been with my family, but I was glad to be back with my husband in Dallas. More checkups were calling me back into the hospital; and I was scheduled to have a chest Computerized Tomography (CT). In my last chest x-ray, there was an ambiguous spot in the upper left lung field. Nobody told me about that radiological finding until almost one year after it was found. Don't ask me why the doctors never informed me, because your guess is as good as mine.

The CT was a requirement to rule-out the possibility of metastatic lung cancer. When the doctor told me they were following up on a finding from last year, I was shockingly surprised. But again I must say, as a cancer patient I was always under a microscope – like it or not.

I had some vague pain with the movement of my left arm after the radiation therapy and thought the side effects may have been the cause of my pain. Possible damage or burning to the lung tissue might have been accountable for the suspicious spot; in any case, radiation therapy has a reputation of affecting normal organ tissue in its attempt to destroy cancerous cells.

When I did not hear anything from the hospital after a week, I understood no news to be good news, figuring the doctors would surely call a patient as soon as any abnormal finding was discovered on a radiographic image.

I trained myself to live one day at a time and erase unnecessary worries from my life. They never helped. I was set free in positive thought patterns, leaving yesterday behind and focusing on the day at hand. I practiced pushing away the static in my head. With rehearsal breathing, exhaling the bad and inhaling the good, I enjoyed peace of mind.

I knew I was dealing with breast cancer, but the diagnosis did not scare me to death because I was absolutely certain of one thing: the universe had a better plan for me. Though it was challenging to control my thoughts and stop them from drifting to the cruel past or an unknown future, I decided to take charge as a leader of my mind. Meditation was my savior. I practiced staying focused on my breathing, quieting the noise of my thoughts, like training a child to keep silent while in conversation with someone else. Soon I learned how to enjoy every single breath of life and live for the *now*.

I picked up the stack of mail from the counter, and weeded through the junk mail that collected while I was in the Middle East. I found several mailings from the hospital, regularly sent to remind me of my next appointment for follow up. One of the letters was from the hospital financial office.

"This is unusual," I thought.

The hospital's financial authorities wrote to notify me about a "discrepancy" in my documents. As a result, they planned to temporarily postpone my treatments and take me off of their coverage until the matter was resolved.

I thought, "What could possibly be wrong for them to eliminate my only source of treatment? What discrepancy?"

I did not have any other form of health coverage. I could not think of any reason to cause the hospital personnel to suspend my enrollment, much less why my enrollment was ultimately terminated even ten days before the contract dictated in the notification letter. Still in need of follow-up case management, my immediate concern was the continuation of my eligibility for treatment.

"What am I going to do without any form of coverage?" Rushing to find out, I called the financial office at the hospital and made an appointment to speak with an administrator.

The waiting room in the hospital, as always, was filled with chattering people – almost none of them English speaking. As if trying to fit into a dress that morphed my form, I felt completely out of place. I sat reading a book, trying to fill the time until I heard my name called. I was asked to bring all of my financial statements from the past six months to date, including our mortgage statements, bank statements and receipts, as well as my passport.

"Why does the hospital want to see my passport?" I wondered.

Interesting question, isn't it?

I could not wait to find out their reasoning.

The financial coordinator called me into her office to tell me, "You have been reported by the breast oncology department. They requested a detailed investigation of your background."

"What do you mean?" I asked.

"We normally don't dig into people's lives unless there is a suspicion. An anonymous person reported your case from the breast oncology ward requesting a thorough investigation about your financial situation. There may be a discrepancy of some sort interfering with your qualifications for the county hospital financial program." She stated.

I could not comprehend what was happening. I lived a life of pride and dignity; and at that moment I did not feel formality was on my side. There I sat on the other side of her desk, nearly through with all of my cancer treatment, my bank account just about empty, and worst of all accused of possible fraudulent activity – politely referred to as a "discrepancy."

In my head, I shuffled through the logs of conversations I held during my numerous visits to the breast oncology clinic. I recalled a mental record of my interactions with all of the doctors and all of the doctor's staff and all of the nurses, etc. Most of them knew I was an unemployed doctor when I entered for treatment, and some became acquainted with my journeys around the world with my husband. As a matter of fact, I remembered sharing with the nurse and intern about my recent trip to visit my family in the Middle East; but I never mentioned to them that my older sister paid for the expenses of my travel. I didn't see its relevance.

I asked myself again, "Why is the financial office in a hospital asking for my passport? They know I am a U.S. citizen." My citizenship was explicitly detailed in my application. I nearly went out of my mind rummaging for an answer.

The scenario that came into my exhausted mind was: "Okay, if I was a staff member in the hospital clinic treating a patient like me, a doctor with a foreign accent, who travels to various borders of the world with her husband, I would likely be asking what the hell is this woman doing in our county hospital designed to treat under-financed patients?"

Of course I couldn't expect everyone to know my entire life story, including my recent financial plummet and hardship. But then again, how does their judgmental mind jump to a conclusive accusation of fraud?

The hospital financial department stopped my coverage without giving me the benefit of the doubt ten days before the coverage would be expired. From their conviction of my case being fraud, I was unfairly scrutinized. From that day forward, each day of going to the hospital was an embarrassment, as if going to the hospital in the first place was not deleterious enough to my soul. I continued going to the hospital as I was scheduled for follow up treatments and was personally billed for each visit or treatment.

"I am not a phony, nor a law-breaker, and I don't want to be made to feel as if I am," I thought.

Each visit I arrived two hours prior to my scheduled appointment in the attempt of resolving the discrepancy.

My credibility as a human was at stake, and their accusations hung around me like a raincloud. I didn't think financial issues or even sickness were on the same level as the credence of ones dignity and pride. Never a day in my life have I felt so insulted and belittled, not even the day I was diagnosed with the breast cancer.

"Lord have mercy!"

I really tried staying calm and collected during my first meeting with the financial department. But my discontentment came out in tears I could not control, streaming down my face, my breathing and speech interrupted by deep sighs.

A week into the investigation, an agent from the hospital police department called us on the telephone. I was so furious, I nearly went postal.

"What do they want from us? Do they think we are some kind of criminals?" I railed on Tom.

"We have done nothing wrong, Sweetheart." Thank goodness my husband was very calm. "This too will pass, like every other bad experiences."

An investigator in the hospital police department separately interviewed my husband and then me. We provided every single piece of paperwork they requested. My fear was that justice would not be served to us; that somehow they would not believe us.

Isn't it true that people have been charged guilty without actually *being* guilty of any charge? For sure there are recorded court cases where people were imprisoned with a life sentence, and later – after spending the better part of their life behind bars – found NOT guilty. I already felt incarcerated by cancer; I wanted to be liberated from this unbearably ugly accusation and move forward.

If we lost the case, we would have to pay every cent of the hospital bill, which had accrued to a mighty large six digit figure. More importantly we would have been stamped with the stigmatism of committing fraud. In fact we were already labeled by our appearance and personal representation; the fraud was actually cast upon us.

Yes indeed, Tom and I were fortunate enough to travel all over the world and enjoy a wonderful life of luxury at one point in time. It seemed a lifetime ago, lo before my illness. Having a house and a car should not constitute grounds to disqualify an individual of having health assistance.

Tom suggested that we sell the house and use the earnings to fund the cost of my remaining treatment. However willing he was, the housing market sunk to an all time low in recent history, and the true value of our home was more than we would be able to ask as a selling price. Rather than helping us, selling the house would have only created more issues. Where would we live? We sought solutions, not more complications.

Health, finance, and now credibility were all together on the line. Keeping faith, we continued to support and love one another. Our love grew deeper and taller through the rain.

During my treatment, Tom kept lots of things a secret to protect my emotions and me. He found me vulnerable and pretended everything was fine. I never knew about the unpaid bills or that he was unemployed. To put my worries at ease, he told me he had a part time job that never actually existed.

Luckily, we were ardently supported and kept afloat by our family and friends. There were records of the deposits into our accounts in amounts that could seem unbelievable to those investigating our case. In Tom's past, he was in a position to financially assist others and to help business acquaintances find job placements. Never did either of us imagine we'd be in need of return favors, nor did we expect them. God shined down upon us with good will, and many people came to our sides to rescue us in our time of need. We are still paying back loans of kindness. The best type of credit is a credit earned when people trust you with their money.

When the investigator interviewed me, I told her Tom and I did not come from a poor background, but many circumstances in our lives delivered us there. I remember telling her, "You know I have cancer and if I am meant to die tomorrow, I don't want to carry a bag of guilt with me by committing fraud for the sake of saving my life."

The qualities of life once thought precious worked against us.

The investigator in the hospital police department examined our case for over a month. Despite our true innocence, sorting through the allegations to reveal the facts of our matter had to have been as difficult as turning around a steam ship in a narrow canal.

One day, after his meeting with the investigator, Tom returned from the hospital with a bouquet of flowers. Wearing a big smile, he reported, "We are cleared and the charges against us are dropped!"

Like the crisp freshness of a lovely spring morning, we became whole again. The police investigator allowed us to recognize that decent and caring people still existed in a world full of judgment. The hospital realized I was a doctor in need of using public services, an honorable citizen just like other existing patients. I wouldn't have wanted to continue as a patient if I was thought to be a fraud.

In retrospect, the investigator was angel-like, and perhaps was God-sent to challenge our poise, and then rescue us from being misjudged. It was a positive turnaround.

14
Scar of Health

E very morning when I am in front of the mirror to apply makeup and change my cloths, I see a scar. My scar is a good sign because it reassures me the tumor is gone. Not too bad of a bargain for earning my life back. The scar also serves as a reminder not to underestimate an enemy. I took care of myself to the best of my ability. Every cancer patient you may talk with will say they have been changed and they are answering cancers' wake-up call to life. It is true. I am one who has been awakened.

What element of being makes a person initiate change? For everyone it may be different, but I think people are propelled by some cause to acknowledge an enhanced dimension to existence.

Upon the realization that our physical body is vulnerable and perishable, the search begins to find a deeper meaning for living. Our physical body is not here to stay forever. Perhaps after suffering, people sense there is only a thin line bordering life from death and are prompted to find the part of themselves that will live on forever. That is to say, the mind and body seek a connection with the higher self, or soul if you will. With the triad united, we are delivered into an enlightened lucidity of wholeness.

With inner focus, I unified my thoughts with my higher self and became genuinely stronger from within. I plugged into the real me – instead of the reflection I saw in the mirror. I pushed aside my physical ailments and tapped into my source of energy coming from a magnetic field encircled around me comprised of spirit and soul.

I don't know exactly how to explain how this phenomenon occurred, but I am a survivor. I found my will. Not only did I have unearthing revelations as a result of the process of being a cancer patient, I also rescued myself from feeling lost in an ocean of problems and self-made obligations that came from an unfulfilled wanting that never ended.

At the start, I did not know who I was as a person. Maybe I was a woman with an ego so big that it tainted my own high expectations of myself and blinded me from seeing others in their true light. I used to think some people were neither as good as me nor good enough for me. I screened people with my criticisms. Having lived through the scrutiny of being misjudged, I no longer judge others.

Today I have the courage to reveal and acknowledge my imperfections. I admit when I need to change, and will.

The peace that comes from spiritual growth is priceless. I feel more in tune with the universe and its beauty. I was physically hurt by cancer but healed spiritually by cancer, ultimately the highest price I had to pay for learning life lessons.

My experience taught me to create positive thought patterns by vocalizing affirmations. I discarded old thought patterns, meaning the constant thoughts of worries and what might happen to me tomorrow. That pattern was a set back to my progress. Now, I am taking one baby step at a time and enjoying my life as it comes to me.

Mind power plays a phenomenal role in our lives. I used my mind as a positive tool to influence my healing abilities. As of today, I still operate with this certified approach towards life. Every day is a brand new day of practicing to stay focused in the present moment, pushing the past or the future away. It is challenging to stop disturbing thoughts of what happened in my past or what might happen in the future. The more I try, the more peace of mind I acquire. I pretty much trained my mind to behave and let me enjoy my life for now. The past is in the past and who knows about the future? Yes, I have plans for my future like everybody else; but I don't like to be preoccupied by possibilities I have no control over.

It is said that time is the best solution to forget about whatever happens in our lives. Forgetting is not entirely the answer though. I don't think about what happened to me, or I should say, I don't allow the shadow of the past to cast darkness onto my life today. On the contrary, I remember every day along my journey for the knowledge I gained. With each step I moved closer to finding myself, and grew into an enhanced approach towards living. My soul is at peace, and I'm more content within my own healthy skin. I have earned this peaceful comfort through disciplined self-training. No one can take that from me. Life is priceless and wonderful. Enjoy!

- THE HAPPY END -

Personal Protocol

As I was going through the process of cancer treatment, this was my personal protocol for healing and creating positive mantras:

Believe in yourself
Meditate daily
Connect with the Universe
Think positive, speak positive
Stay away from negative people; Fill life with loved ones
Manage stress by staying informed & planning
Research before starting treatment
Know all options
Don't be judgmental: it distracts the healthy mind
Eat healthy balanced nutritious meals
Use glassware (not plastic!)
Drink clean, filtered water
Stay active
Walk often
Breathe fresh air
Engage in fun activities
Fill your soul with love
Make a wish list with action steps and walk towards dreams
Be happy and content
Laugh Laugh Laugh
Enjoy every day as if this is your last
I did it, can you? Please do!

"Organic Iron Chef" Recipes

Would you like to join me for lunch? I am not cooking. Tom, our "Organic Iron Chef" performs all the cooking; but don't be fooled, I am still the 'buss-boy' clearing and cleaning the counter-tops! Tom's cooking is so delicious: it is a bite into life. We always purchase organic foods and highly recommend this practice. If you are a cancer patient, please consult your physician or a qualified nutritionist for foods to eat during your treatment and to learn a diet best for you.

Humans have the tendency to forget, which can be quite helpful in some cases. However, I try to remember what I am eating because it has such an enormous effect on who I am. I steer clear of all processed foods, sugars, and trans-fats. To fuel my body's engine, I drive towards fresh, natural, organic, nutritious produce close to the vine of life, and always maintain my fluid levels with proper intake of clean filtered water.

Nutrition is like a religion, and pre-packed, processed canned foods taboo. Today I am free of cancer and celebrating life. What a bumpy road behind us. The "Organic

Iron Chef" and the princess are planning to live happily ever after.

Here are menu choices, organic, low fat and delicious assortments. Remember to lightly steam all fresh vegetables to avoid bacteria.

Recipes

Green field salad with toasted almond

*Serves Two:
½ pack green field salad (pre-washed and packed)
6 to 8 cherry tomatoes: wash thoroughly & slice
1 tbsp chopped basil (dry basil if fresh is not available)
½ of a lime: juiced
2 tbsp extra virgin olive oil
1 clove garlic chopped (or ½ tsp garlic powder)
2 tbsp almonds: toasted

In a small skillet, toast the sliced almonds over low heat; Low sodium salt and freshly ground pepper to your taste. Stir frequently (to avoid burning) and remove from heat when color turns golden/tan. Let almonds cool (you may also toast in advance as a snack and keep stored in a zip lock bag refrigerated). Toss all the ingredients into a serving bowl; serve it in a salad plate and top with toasted almond.

Lentil soup

1 tbsp olive oil
½ tsp cumin powder or seeds
1 tsp turmeric
1tsp low sodium salt
¼ tsp cayenne pepper
1tsp limejuice
1 cup lentil pre soaked
1 small potato diced
1 small onion diced
1 small carrot diced
2 clove garlic diced
2 tbsp chopped cilantro

In a medium saucepan, bring two cups of water to a boil; add all the ingredients except olive oil and cilantro. Let it stand over low-medium heat covered (stir periodically) for ½ hour or until done. Add olive oil and cilantro before serving. Serve hot with a slice of whole grain toast or pita bread.

Baked salmon with pesto sauce

One piece of wild Atlantic Ocean salmon
1 tsp olive oil
1 clove diced garlic
½ tsp turmeric
½ lime juiced
1 tsp low sodium salt
1 tbsp pesto sauce
1 cup steamed vegetables of your choice

Pre heat oven to 375°; and line a baking tray with foil. Wash, rinse and dry the fish. Lightly cover the fish with olive oil, limejuice, sprinkled salt and pepper. Bake for between 15 to 20 minutes (avoid over cooking, it makes the fish dry). top the fish with pesto sauce. Use a side dish of steamed vegetables or salad or even with brown rice.

Dessert

Apple with blue berry sauce.

One gala or Washington apple thickly sliced and cored
½ cup fresh or frozen blue berries
1 tbsp honey
½ tsp cardamom powder
½ tsp vanilla
1-cup water

In a small pot, soak vanilla, cardamom, and apple slices in ½ cup water for 10 minutes; simmer at a low-med heat, covered until apples are semi-soft (insert a tooth pick to check). In a small saucepan, simmer blueberries and honey with ½ cup water until it a thickened syrupy (about 10 minutes). In a shallow serving dish, place cooked apples top with blueberry sauce. Garnish with fresh mint; Serve warm.

My favorite Veggie Juice

5 to 6 large carrots
1 red apple
1 small or ½ medium size skinned beet
½ stem celery
½ tsp freshly diced ginger

Using a juicer, juice all the ingredients. Pour into a jar and let cool in the fridge for ½ hours.

www.2GreenApples.org

Other Books and Products

Adult Potty Training
Organic Iron Chef
Saving Love
Why Not Me? An Inspiring True Story of Survival

Smart Cookies™: The name says it all! Eating right is the key. This homemade Smart Cookie™ has dates and walnuts making for a high-energy snack. Great with a warm drink. Ingredients: organic flour, organic eggs, dates, walnuts, cardamom and grape seed oil. Contains no preservatives, no dairy products, no sugar and is low in fat.

Biscotti: Once you start eating this cookie, you cannot stop! The constructive activity of baking this Italian dipping cookie during her treatment helped Vida keep her mind busy. In addition, the sales of Biscotti have funded *2 Green Apples, Inc.* With every bite of Vida's biscotti, you have a double pleasure of a scrumptious treat and helping a woman in financial need. The triple baked biscotti contains no preservatives, no dairy products, and is low in both fat and sugar.

www.2GreenApples.org

A Kind Word About The Beautiful Author

Vida means to me "ever present" and describes the true essence of my dear friend. Prominent in any crowd, her beauty lights up a room. Vida's imaginative mind explores deeply in search for meaning and purpose not just for herself, but for others, too. She responds to everyone, everything and every event with a gentle and melodious voice of harmony.

Through her physical and metaphysical healing practices she infuses compassion, wisdom, patience and persistence to all that come in contact with her. She is fully present and alive; and her inner spirit radiates with joy and acceptance.

Vida celebrates every breath of life heartily through her talented creativity with painting, music and words. Her passion is to give and to share the perfume of "living;" then, her inner child marvels as she watches her friends bloom into flowers.

-Dr. Heather Hosseini

International Health Publishing
Inspiring and challenging the world to see the light!
Our mission is to create publications exposing the truth,
Encouraging spiritual enlightenment,
Facilitating growth and healing
All while providing a phenomenal experience

International Health Publishing
Little and Growing
(978) 846-1964
www.InternationalHealthPublishing.com

For more information on books and products by
Dr. Vida Meymand and *2 Green Apples, Inc.*
Visit www.2GreenApples.org
www.whynotme.tv